High Throughput Screening

METHODS IN MOLECULAR BIOLOGY™

John M. Walker, SERIES EDITOR

High Throughput Screening

Methods and Protocols

Edited by

William P. Janzen

Amphora Discovery,
Research Triangle Park, NC

Humana Press ✻ **Totowa, New Jersey**

Production Editor: Mark J. Breaugh.
Cover design by Patricia F. Cleary.

For additional copies, pricing for bulk purchases, and/or information about other Humana titles, contact Humana at the above address or at any of the following numbers: Tel.: 973-256-1699; Fax: 973-256-8341; E-mail: humana@humanapr.com or visit our Website: http://humanapress.com

Library of Congress Cataloging in Publication Data

High throughput screening : methods and protocols / edited by William P. Janzen.
    p. cm. -- (Methods in molecular biology ; v. 190)
  Includes bibiographical references and index.
  ISBN 0-89603-889-0 (alk. paper)
  1. High throughput screening (Drug development) I. Janzen, William P. II. Series.

  RS419.5 .H54 2002
615'.19--dc21

Preface

Science is changing. As new methods evolve to generate data and create knowledge from it, the pace of discovery increases on an ever-steeper slope. One of the most fundamental changes is our ability and desire to approach the scientific method on a grander scale. Scientists can no longer afford to carefully isolate a single hypothesis and test it exhaustively before moving on to the next experiment. Now we must intellectually grasp an entire system, design experiments to test its many variables, and then probe them in a single multivariate experiment. Fortunately, innumerable new tools are being developed to facilitate this change.

The field we address in *High Throughput Screening* (HTS) has evolved in the midst of these changes and, I like to think, been instrumental in the creation of many of the enabling tools and methodologies. On the simplest level, HTS is the testing of large numbers of candidate molecules in a biological assay. However, when one considers that, at the time of this writing, large is generally accepted to entail over 500,000 samples in a period of only a few weeks or days, and that those numbers have doubled every two years for the past decade, the perspective changes.

High throughput screening requires the successful integration of four diverse scientific disciplines. The Biological sciences, including Pharmacology, Genomics, Molecular Biology, Enzymology, and Biochemistry, yield the targets and screens. A mastery of Chemistry is required to produce diverse libraries of compounds for testing as well as to optimize the lead compounds. Because of the level of industrialization of HTS, Engineering obviously plays an increasingly important role. Finally, the millions of data points produced must be mined for meaningful knowledge, so Information Technology becomes a lynchpin in the operation. Underlying all these is a need for logistical management and above all, a hunger for speed!

Arguably, the first high throughput screen took place in 1948–1949 when Charles Pfizer and Company organized a team of 56 scientists who examined 100,000 soil samples for antibiotic activity over an 18 month period *(1)*. This effort resulted in the discovery of Terramycin, which eventually captured half of the broad-spectrum antibiotic market—and the race was on. Pharmaceutical, chemical, and agricultural companies amassed collections (libraries) of chemical compounds from their efforts that were then reused in other discovery efforts. With the advent of laboratory robotics in the 1990s, it became feasible to test these libraries in their entirety in screening targets and the field of HTS came into its own.

Although HTS has become an integral part of nearly every discovery operation, there is not a clear career path into the field or an associated body of literature. Until recently, nearly every scientist working in HTS had a unique story detailing precisely how they had arrived there. All that is changing. Training programs are beginning to appear and the techniques created in HTS are being used more and more frequently in laboratories outside the field. By providing both background material and real-use cases of HTS technology, I hope this manual will serve as an introduction for those seeking a greater understanding of HTS, as well as provide enough detail to be useful for scientists in established lead generation laboratories. Each author was asked to submit the chapter they wished they had been provided at the time they started in HTS. I hope that their efforts will be of use to you.

I would like to thank Celestine Pulliam, LouAnn Mitchell, and Wendy Spencer for their assistance in the preparation of this volume.

William P. Janzen

Reference

1. Sneader, Walter (1985) Drug Discovery: The Evolution of Modern Medicines. John Wiley and Sons, New York, NY.

Contents

vii

Contributors

LAURA ABRIOLA • *Novartis Pharmaceuticals Corporation, Summit, NJ*

MELVYN BAEZ • *Lilly Research Laboratories, Eli Lilly and Company, Indianapolis, IN*

DOUGLAS S. BURDETTE • *Pfizer Global Research and Development, Ann Arbor, MI*

JOHN W. CARPENTER • *Sphinx Laboratories, Eli Lilly and Company, Research Triangle Park, NC*

JAMES A. CHAN • *Department of Molecular Screening, GlaxoSmithKline, King of Prussia, PA*

SETH COHEN • *Millenium Pharmaceuticals Inc., Cambridge, MA*

THOMAS K. ECKOLS • *Sphinx Laboratories, Eli Lilly and Company, Research Triangle Park, NC*

DAVID A. GIEGEL • *Pfizer Global Research and Development, Ann Arbor, MI*

STEVEN HAMILTON • *Sanitas Consulting, Boulder, CO*

ROBERT P. HERTZBERG • *Department of Molecular Screening, GlaxoSmithKline, King of Prussia, PA*

FREDERICK R. HUBBARD • *Sphinx Laboratories, Eli Lilly and Company, Research Triangle Park, NC*

JUAN A. HUESO-RODRÍGUEZ • *Department of Molecular Screening, GlaxoSmithKline, Madrid, Spain*

BARBARA HYND • *Private Practice, West Chester, OH*

WILLIAM P. JANZEN • *Amphora Discovery, Research Triangle Park, NC*

PATRICIA JOHNSTON • *Sphinx Laboratories, Eli Lilly and Company, Research Triangle Park, NC*

PAUL A. JOHNSTON • *Sphinx Laboratories, Eli Lilly and Company, Research Triangle Park, NC*

WILMA W. KEIGHLEY • *Lead Discovery Technologies, Pfizer Global R&D, Sandwich, UK*

CARMEN LAETHEM • *Sphinx Laboratories, Eli Lilly and Company, Research Triangle Park, NC*

SUSAN E. LOWE • *Bristol-Myers Squibb Pharmaceutical Research Institute, Wallingford, CT*

RICARDO MACARRÓN • *Department of Molecular Screening, GlaxoSmithKline, King of Prussia, PA*

SUSAN P. MANLY • *Bristol-Myers Squibb Pharmaceutical Research Institute, Wallingford, CT*

JAMES S. MARKS • *Pfizer Global Research and Development, Ann Arbor, MI*

DON MCCLURE • *Lilly Research Laboratories, Eli Lilly and Company, Indianapolis, IN*

KARL C. MENKE • *Sphinx Laboratories, Eli Lilly and Company, Research Triangle Park, NC*

DAVID L. G. NELSON • *Lilly Research Laboratories, Eli Lilly and Company, Indianapolis, IN*

RAMESH PADMANABHA • *Bristol-Myers Squibb Pharmaceutical Research Institute, Wallingford, CT*

ROBERT H. SCHWEITZER • *Novartis Pharmaceuticals Corporation, Summit, NJ*

ROBERT F. TRINKA • *American Diagnostica Inc., Greenwich, CT*

TERRY P. WOOD • *Lead Discovery Technologies, Pfizer Global R&D, Sandwich, UK*

JINZI J. WU • *Immunex Corporation, Seattle, WA*

1

Design and Implementation of High Throughput Screening Assays

Ricardo Macarrón and Robert P. Hertzberg

1. Introduction

In most pharmaceutical and biotechnology companies, high throughput screening (HTS) is a central function in the drug-discovery process. This has resulted from the fact that there are increasing numbers of validated therapeutic targets being discovered through advances in human genomics, and increasing numbers of chemical compounds being produced through high-throughput chemistry initiatives. Many large companies study 100 targets or more each year, and in order to progress these targets, lead compounds must be found. Increasingly, pharmaceutical companies are relying on HTS as the primary engine driving lead discovery.

The HTS process is a subset of the drug discovery process and can be described as the phase from Target to Lead. This phase can be broken down in the following steps:

Target Choice
⇓
Reagent Procurement ⇔ Assay Development and Validation
⇓
Screening Collections ⇒HTS Implementation
⇓
Data Capture, Storage and Analysis
⇓
Leads

It is critically important to align the target choice and assay method to ensure that a biologically relevant and robust screen is configured. Every screening

From: *Methods in Molecular Biology, vol. 190: High Throughput Screening: Methods and Protocols*
Edited by: W. P. Janzen © Humana Press Inc., Totowa, NJ

laboratory can relate stories of assays being delivered that are incompatible with modern robotic screening instruments and unacceptable in terms of signal to background or variability. To avoid this problem, organizations must ensure that communication between therapeutic departments, assay-development groups, and screening scientists occurs early, as soon as the target is chosen, and throughout the assay-development phase.

Reagent procurement is often a major bottleneck in the HTS process. This can delay the early phases of assay development, e.g., when active protein cannot be obtained, and also delay HTS implementation if scale-up of protein or cells fails to produce sufficient reagent to run the full screen. For efficient HTS operation, there must be sufficient reagent available to run the entire screening campaign before production HTS can start. Otherwise, the campaign will need to stop halfway through and the screening robots will have to be reconfigured for other work. Careful scheduling between reagent procurement departments and HTS functions is critical to ensure optimum use of robotics and personnel. To improve scheduling, modern HTS laboratories are moving toward a supply-chain model similar to that used in industrial factories.

Successful HTS implementation is multidisciplinary and requires close alignment of personnel maintaining and distributing screening collections, technology specialists responsible for setting up and supporting HTS automation, biologists and biochemists with knowledge of assay methodology, information technology (IT) personnel capable of collecting and analyzing large data sets, and chemists capable of examining screening hits to look for patterns that define lead series. Through the marriage of these diverse specialties, therapeutic targets can be put through the lead discovery engine called HTS and lead compounds will emerge.

2. Choice of Therapeutic Target

While disease relevance should be the main driver when choosing a therapeutic target, one should also consider factors important to the HTS process. These factors are technical, i.e. whether a statistically robust and sufficiently simple assay can be configured, as well as chemical. Chemical considerations relate to the probability that compounds capable of producing the therapeutically relevant effect against a specific target are: 1) present in the screening collection, 2) can be found through screening, and 3) have drug-like physicochemical properties.

Years of experience in HTS within the industry have suggested that certain targets are more 'chemically tractable' than others. Recent studies of top-selling prescription drugs have shown that G-protein coupled receptors (GPCRs), ion channels, nuclear hormone receptors and proteases are among the most exploitable target classes, i.e., drugs against these targets produce the highest sales. Among these targets, GPCRs are normally thought of as the most chemically tractable, since there are more GPCR drugs on the market than drugs for any other target class. Furthermore, evidence indicates that HTS campaigns against GPCRs produce lead compounds at a higher rate than many other target classes *(1)*. Kinases are another chemically tractable class that often affords lead compounds from screening (*see* Chapter 4); however, while many kinase inhibitors are in clinical trials, none have yet reached the market.

On the other side of the spectrum, targets that work via protein-protein interactions have a lower probability of being successful in HTS campaigns. One reason for this is the fact that compound libraries often do not contain compounds of sufficient size and complexity to disrupt the large surface of protein-protein interaction that is encountered in these targets. Natural products are one avenue that may be fruitful against protein-protein targets, since these compounds are often larger and more complex than those in traditional chemical libraries (*see* Chapter 9). The challenge for these targets is finding compounds that have the desired inhibitory effect and also contain drug-like properties (e.g., are not too large in molecular weight). Recently, several groups have begun to tackle this problem by screening for small fragments that inhibit the interaction and joining them together to produce moderate-sized potent inhibitors.

Certain subsets of protein-protein interaction targets have been successful from an HTS point of view. For example, chemokines receptors are technically a protein-protein interaction (within the GPCR class) and there are several examples of successful lead compounds for targets in this class *(2)*. Similarly, certain integrin receptors that rely on small epitopes (i.e., RGD sequences) have also been successful at producing lead compounds *(3)*. There may be other classes of tractable protein-protein interactions that remain undiscovered due to limitations in compound libraries.

Based on the thinking that chemically tractable targets are easier to inhibit, most pharmaceutical companies have concentrated much of their effort on these targets and diminished work on more difficult targets. While this approach makes sense from a cost-vs-benefit point of view, one should be careful not to eliminate entirely target classes that would otherwise be extremely attractive from a biological point of view. Otherwise, the prophecy of chemical tractability will be self-fulfilled, since today's compound collections will not expand into new regions and we will never find leads for more difficult biologically relevant targets. There is clearly an important need for enhancing collections by filling holes that chemical history has left open. The challenge is filling these holes with drug-like compounds that are different from the traditional pharmacophores of the past.

A second and equally important factor to consider when choosing targets is the technical probability of developing a robust and high-quality screening assay. The impact of new assay technologies has made this less important, since there are now many good assay methods available for a wide variety of target types (*see* **Subheading 3.**). Nevertheless, some targets are more technically difficult than others. Of the target types mentioned earlier, GPCRs, kinases, proteases, nuclear hormone receptors, and protein-protein interactions are often relatively easy to establish screens for. Ion channels are more difficult, although new technologies are being developed that make these more approachable from an HTS point of view *(4)*. Enzymes other than kinases and proteases must be considered on a case-by-case basis depending on the nature of the substrates involved.

Reagent procurement is also a factor to consider, obtaining sufficient reagents for the screening campaign can sometimes be time-consuming, expensive, and unpredictable. In the case of protein target, this depends on the ease with which the particular protein(s) can be expressed and purified; the amount of protein needed per screening test; and the commercial cost of any substrates, ligands, or consumables.

All of these factors must be considered on a case-by-case basis and should be evaluated at the beginning of a Target-to-Lead effort before making a choice to go forward. Working on an expensive and technically difficult target must be balanced against the degree of validation and biological relevance. While the perfect target is chemically tractable, technically easy, inexpensive, fully validated, and biologically relevant, such targets are rare. The goal is to work on a portfolio that spreads the risk among these factors and balances the available resources.

3. Choice of Assay Method

There are usually several ways of looking for hits of any given target. The first and major choice to make is between a biochemical or a cell-based assay (*see* Chapter 6). By biochemical we understand an assay developed to look for compounds that interact with an isolated target in an artificial environment. This has been the most popular approach in the early 1990s, the decade in which HTS became a mature and central area of drug discovery. This bias toward biochemical assays for HTS is partly driven by the fact that cell-based assays are often more difficult to run in high throughput. However, recent advances in technology and instrumentation for cell-based assays have occurred over the past few years. Among these is the emergence of HTS-compatible technology to measure GPCR *(5)* and ion channel function *(4)*, confocal imaging platforms for rapid cellular and subcellular imaging, and the continued development of reporter-gene technology.

3.1. Biochemical Assay Methods

While laborious separation-based assay formats such as radiofiltration and enzyme-linked immunosorbent assays (ELISAs) were common in the early 1990s, most biochemical screens in use today use simple homogeneous "mix-and-read" formats (Chapter 3 provides more details). These technologies— including scintillation proximity assay (SPA), fluorescence intensity (FLINT), fluorescence polarization (FP), fluorescence resonance energy transfer (FRET), time-resolved energy transfer (TRET) and others—are now the workhorses of the modern HTS laboratory *(6)*.

The most common assay readouts used in biochemical assay methods for HTS are optical, including scintillation, fluorescence, absorbance, and luminescence. Among these, fluorescence-based techniques are among the most important detection approaches used for HTS. Fluorescence techniques give very high sensitivity, which allows assay miniaturization, and are amenable to homogeneous formats. One factor to consider when developing fluorescence assays for screening compound collections is wavelength; in general, short excitation wavelengths (especially those below 400 nm) should be avoided to minimize interference produced by test compounds.

Although fluorescence intensity measurements have been successfully applied in HTS, this format is mostly applied to a narrow range of enzyme targets for which fluorogenic substrates are available. A more versatile fluorescence technique is FP, which can be used to measure bimolecular association events *(7)*. Many examples of HTS applications of FP have now been reported, including ligand-receptor binding and enzyme assays in 1536-well plates. Another important fluorescence readout is TRET *(7)*. This is a dual-labeling approach that is based on long-range energy transfer between fluorescent Ln^{3+}-complexes and a suitable resonance-energy acceptor. These approaches give high sensitivity by reducing background, and a large number of HTS assays have now been configured using TRET. This technique is highly suited to measurements of protein-protein interactions.

One area of fluorescence spectroscopy that is just starting to be applied to HTS is that of single-molecule fluctuation-based measurements. These methods are performed using confocal optics in which the observation volume is extremely small (~ 1 fL). The classical form of confocal fluctuation spectroscopy, known as fluorescence correlation spectroscopy (FCS), has now been demonstrated to be a viable approach to HTS *(7,8)*. Fluorescence intensity distribution analysis (FIDA), a related method for analyzing fluctuation data that may be more versatile than FCS, involves the measurement of molecular brightness within a confocal observation volume *(8)*.

While fluorescence assay technologies are growing in importance, current estimates from various surveys of HTS laboratories indicate that radiometric assays presently constitute between 20 and 50% of all screens performed. Important radiometric techniques include scintillation proximity techniques such as SPA/Leadseeker™ (Amersham Pharmacia Biotech, Cardiff, Wales) and FlashPlates™ (NEN Life Science Products, Boston, MA). These techniques have been used for a wide variety of applications including kinases, nucleic acid-processing enzymes, ligand-receptor interactions, and detection of cAMP levels *(6)*. Of course, radiometric assays have several disadvantages including safety, limited reagent stability, relatively long read-times, and little intrinsic information on the isotope environment. However, imaging plate readers are now emerging to address the issue of read-time and assay miniaturization.

3.2. Cell-based Assay Methods (see also Chapter 6)

As recently as the mid-1990s, most cell-based assay formats were not consistent with HTS requirements. However, as recent technological advances have facilitated higher throughput functional assays, cell-based formats now make up a reasonable proportion of screens performed today. The FLIPR™ (Molecular Devices, Sunnyvale, CA) is a fluorescence imaging plate reader with integrated liquid handling that facilitates the simultaneous fluorescence imaging of 384 samples to measure intracellular calcium mobilization in real time *(5)*. This format is now commonly used for GPCR and ion channel targets. Another promising technology for ion channels is based on voltage-sensitive fluorescence resonance energy transfer (VIPR™; Aurora Biosciences, La Jolla, CA) *(4)*.

The reporter gene assay is another common cell-based format amenable to HTS. This method offers certain advantages over FLIPR™ and VIPR™, in that it requires fewer cells, is easier to automate and can be performed in 1536-well plates. Recent descriptions of miniaturized reporter gene readouts include luciferase, secreted alkaline phosphate, and beta-lactamase. Another cell-based screening format based on cell darkening in frog melanophores has been applied to screening for GPCR and other receptor targets *(6)*.

Recently, imaging systems have been developed that quantify cellular and subcellular fluorescence in whole cells. These systems have the capability of bringing detailed assays with high information content into the world of HTS. One of the most advanced systems is the ArrayScan™ (Cellomics, Pittsburgh, PA), which has been used to measure GPCR internalization as well as a range of other applications *(6)*.

3.3. Matching Assay Method to Target Type

Often, one has a choice of assay method for a given target type (**Table 1**). To illustrate the various factors that are important when choosing an assay type, let's consider the important GPCR target class. GPCRs can be screened using cell-based assays such as FLIPR and reporter gene; or biochemical formats such as SPA, FP, or FIDA. One overriding factor when choosing between functional or binding assays for GPCRs is whether one seeks to find agonists or antagonists. Functional assays such as FLIPR and reporter gene are much more amenable to finding agonists than are binding assays, while antagonists can be found with either format. FLIPR assays are relatively easy to develop, but this screening method is labor-intensive (particularly with respect to cell-culture requirements) and more difficult to automate than reporter-gene assays. In contrast, the need for longer-term incubation times for reporter-gene assays (4–6 h vs min for FLIPR) means that cytotoxic interference by test compounds may be more problematic. On the plus side, reporter-gene readouts for GPCRs can sometimes be more sensitive to agonists than FLIPR.

Regarding biochemical assays for GPCRs, SPA is the most common format since radiolabeling is often facile and nonperturbing. However, fluorescence assays for GPCRs such as FP and FIDA are becoming more important. Fluorescent labels are more stable, safer, and often more economical than radiolabels. However, while fluorescent labeling is becoming easier and more predictable, these labels are larger and thus can sometimes perturb the biochemical interaction (in either direction).

In general, one should choose the assay format that is easiest to develop, most predictable, most relevant, and easiest to run. These factors, however, are not always known in advance. And even worse, they can be at odds with each other and thus must be balanced to arrive at the best option. In some cases, it makes sense to parallel track two formats during the assay-development phase and choose between them based on which is easiest to develop and most facile. Finally, in addition to these scientific considerations, logistical factors such as the number of specific readers or robot types available in the HTS lab and the queue size for these systems must be taken into account.

4. Assay Development and Validation

The final conditions of an HTS assay are chosen following the optimization of quality without compromising throughput, while keeping costs low. The most critical points that must be considered in the design of a high-quality assay are biochemical data and statistical performance. Achieving an accept-

Table 1
The Most Important Assay Formats for Various Target Types

Target type	Assay formats	
	Biochemical	Cell-based
GPCRs	SPA, FP, FIDA	FLIPR, reporter gene, melanophores
Ion channels		FLIPR, VIPR
Nuclear hormone receptor	FP, TRET, SPA	Reporter gene
Kinases	FP, TRET, SPA	
Protease	FLINT, FRET, FP, SPA	Reporter gene
Other enzymes	FLINT, FRET, FP, SPA, TRET, colorimetry	
Protein-protein	TRET, BET, SPA	Reporter gene

able performance while keeping assay conditions within the desired range often requires an assay-optimization step. This usually significantly improves the stability and/or activity of the biological system studied, and has therefore become a key step in the development of screening assays.

4.1. Critical Biochemical Parameters in HTS Assays

The success of an HTS campaign in finding hits of the desired profile depends primarily on the presence of such compounds in the collection tested. But it is also largely dependent on the ability of the researcher to engineer the assay in accordance with that profile while reaching an appropriate statistical performance.

A classical example that illustrates the importance of the assay design is how substrate concentration determines the sensitivity for different kind of enzymatic inhibitors. If we set the concentration of one substrate in a screening assay at $10 \times$ Km, competitive inhibitors of that enzyme-substrate interaction with a Ki greater than 1/11 of the compound concentration used in HTS will show less than 50% inhibition and will likely be missed; i.e., competitive inhibitors with a Ki of 0.91 μM or higher would be missed when screening at 10 μM. On the other hand, the same problem will take place for uncompetitive inhibitors if substrate concentration is set at 1/10 of its Km. Therefore, it is important to know what kind of hits are sought in order to make the right choices in substrate concentration; often, one chooses a substrate concentration that facilitates discovery of both competitive and uncompetitive inhibitors.

In this section, we describe the biochemical parameters of an assay that have a greater influence on the sensitivity of finding different classes of hits and some recommendations about where to set them.

4.1.1. Enzymatic Assays

4.1.1.1. Substrate Concentration

The sensitivity of an enzymatic assay to different types of inhibitors is a function of the ratio of substrate concentration to Km (S/Km).

- Competitive inhibitors: for reversible inhibitors that bind to a binding site that is the same as one substrate, the more of that substrate present in the assay, the less inhibition will be observed. The relationship between IC_{50} (compound concentration required to observe 50% inhibition of enzymatic activity with respect to an uninhibited control) and Ki (inhibition constant) is (9):

$$IC_{50} = (1 + S/Km) \times Ki$$

As shown in **Fig. 1**, at S/Km ratios less than 1 the assay is more sensitive to competitive inhibitors, with an asymptotic limit of IC_{50} = Ki. At high S/Km ratios, the assay becomes less suitable for finding this type of inhibitors.

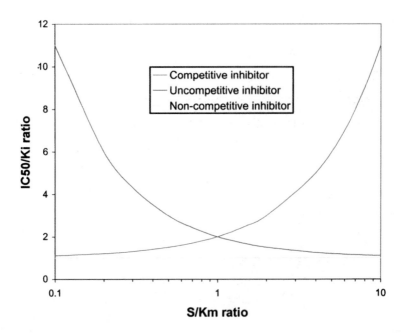

Fig. 1. Variation of IC_{50}/Ki ratio with the S/Km ratio for different type of inhibitors. At [S] = Km, IC_{50} = 2Ki for competitive (blue line) and uncompetitive (red line) inhibitors. For non-competitive inhibitors (yellow line) IC_{50} = Ki at all substrate concentrations.

- Uncompetitive inhibitors: if the inhibitor binds to the enzyme-substrate complex or any other intermediate complex but not to the free enzyme, the dependence on S/Km is the opposite to what has been described for competitive binders. The relationship between IC_{50} and Ki is (**9**):

$$IC_{50} = (1 + Km/S) \times Ki$$

  High substrate concentrations make the assay more sensitive to uncompetitive inhibitors (**Fig. 1**).

- Noncompetitive (allosteric) inhibitors: if the inhibitor binds with equal affinity to the free enzyme and to the enzyme-substrate complex, the inhibition observed is independent of the substrate concentration. The relationship between IC_{50} and Ki is (**9**):

$$IC_{50} = Ki$$

- Mixed inhibitors: if the inhibitor binds to the free enzyme and to the enzyme-substrate complex with different affinities (Ki1 and Ki2, respectively), the relationship between IC_{50} and Ki is (**10**):

$$IC_{50} = (S + Km)/(Km/Ki1 + S/Ki2)$$

Table 2
Examples of Limitations to Substrate Concentration
Imposed by Some Popular Assay Technologies

Assay Technology	Limitations[a]
Fluorescence	Inner filter effect at high concentrations of fluorophore (usually $> 1\ \mu M$)
Fluorescence polarization	>30% substrate depletion required
Capture techniques (ELISA, SPA, FlashPlate, BET, others)	Concentrations of the reactant captured must be in alignment with the upper limit of binding capacity.
Capture techniques and anyone monitoring binding	Nonspecific binding (NSB) of the product or of any reactant to the capture element (bead, plate, membrane, antibody, etc.) may result in misleading activity determinations
All	Sensitivity limits impose a lower limit to the amount of product detected

[a]These limitations also apply to ligand in binding assays or other components in assays monitoring any kind of binding event.

In summary, setting the substrate(s) concentration(s) at the Km value is an optimal way of ensuring that all type of inhibitors exhibiting a Ki close to or below the compound concentration in the assay can be found in an HTS campaign. Nevertheless, if there is a specific interest in favoring or avoiding a certain type of inhibitor, then the S/Km ratio would be chosen considering the information provided earlier. For instance, many ATP-binding enzymes are tested in the presence of saturating concentrations of ATP to minimize inhibition from compounds that bind to the ATP-binding site.

Quite often the cost of one substrate or the limitations of the technique used to monitor enzymatic activity (**Table 2**) may preclude setting the substrate concentration at its ideal point.

As in many other situations found while implementing a HTS assay, the screening scientist must consider all factors involved and look for the optimal solution. For instance, if the sensitivity of a detection technology requires setting S = 10 × Km to achieve an acceptable signal to background, competitive inhibitors with a Ki greater than 1/11 of the compound concentration tested will not be found and will limit the campaign to finding more potent inhibitors. In this case, working at a higher compound concentration would help to find some of the weak inhibitors otherwise missed. If this is not feasible, it is better to lose weak inhibitors while running a statistically robust assay, rather than making the assay more sensitive by lowering substrate concentration to a point of unacceptable signal to background. The latter approach is riskier since a bad

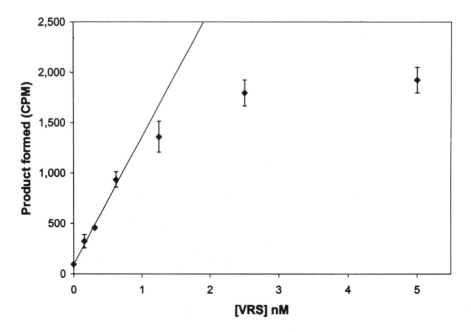

Fig. 2. Protein dilution curve for valyl-tRNA synthetase. The activity was measured after 20 min incubation following the SPA procedure described *(11)*.

statistical performance would jeopardize the discovery of more potent hits (*see* **Subheading 4.3.**).

4.1.1.2. ENZYME CONCENTRATION

The accuracy of inhibition values calculated from enzymatic activity in the presence of inhibitors relies on the linear response of activity to the enzyme concentration. Therefore, an enzyme dilution study must be performed in order to determine the linear range of enzymatic activity with respect to enzyme concentration.

As shown in **Fig. 2** for valyl-tRNA synthetase, at high enzyme concentrations there is typically a loss of linearity due to either substrate depletion, protein aggregation, or limitations in the detection system. If the enzyme is not stable at low concentrations, or if the assay method does not respond linearly to product formation or substrate depletion, there could also be a lack of linearity in the lower end.

In addition, enzyme concentration marks a lower limit to the accurate determination of inhibitor potency. IC_{50} values lower than one half of the enzyme concentration cannot be measured; this effect is often referred to as "bottoming out." As the quality of compound collections improves, this could be a real problem since structure activity relationship (SAR) trends cannot be observed among the more potent hits. Obviously, enzyme concentration must be kept far below the concentration of compounds tested in order to find any inhibitor. In general, compounds are tested at micromolar concentrations (1–100 μ*M*) and, as a rule of thumb, it is advisable to work at enzyme concentrations below 100 n*M*.

On the other hand, the assay can be made insensitive to certain undesired hits (such as inhibitors of enzymes added in coupled systems) by using higher concentrations of these proteins. In any case, the limiting step of a coupled system must be the one of interest, and thus the auxiliary enzymes should always be in excess.

4.1.1.3. INCUBATION TIME AND DEGREE OF SUBSTRATE DEPLETION

As described earlier for enzyme concentration, it is important to assess the linearity vs time of the reaction analyzed. Most HTS assays are end-point and so it is crucial to select an appropriate incubation time. Although linearity vs enzyme concentration is not achievable if the end-point selected does not lie in the linear range of the progress curves for all enzyme concentrations involved, exceptions to this rule do happen, and so it is important to check it as well.

To determine accurate kinetic constants, it is crucial to measure initial velocities. However, for the determination of acceptable inhibition values it is sufficient to be close to linearity. Therefore, the classical rule found in biochemistry textbooks of working at or below 10% substrate depletion (e.g., **ref. *12***) does not necessarily apply to HTS assays. Provided that all compounds in a collection are treated in the same way, if the inhibitions observed are off by a narrow margin it is not a problem. As shown in **Fig. 3**, at 50% substrate depletion with an initial substrate concentration at its Km, the inhibition observed for a 50% real inhibition is 45%, an acceptable error. For higher inhibitions the errors are lower (e.g. instead of 75% inhibition 71% would be observed). At lower S/Km ratios the errors are slightly higher (e.g., at S = 1/10 Km, a 50% real inhibition would yield an observed 4 % inhibition, again at 50% substrate depletion).

This flexibility to work under close-to-linearity but not truly linear reaction rates makes it feasible to use certain assay technologies in HTS, e.g., fluorescence polarization, that require a high proportion of substrate depletion in order to produce a significant change in signal. Secondary assays configured within linear rates should allow a more accurate determination of IC$_{50}$s for hits.

In reality, the experimental progress curve for a given enzyme may differ from the theoretical one depicted here for various reasons such as non-Michaelis-Menten behavior, reagent deterioration, inhibition by product, detection artifacts, etc. In view of the actual progress curve, practical choices should be made to avoid missing interesting hits.

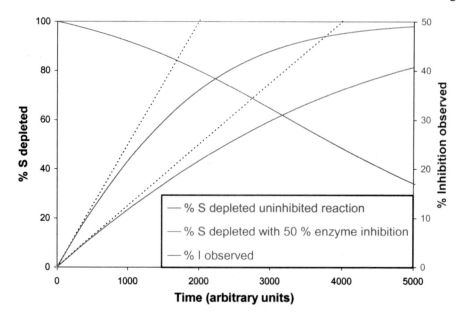

Fig. 3. Theoretical progress curves at S = Km of an uninhibited enzymatic reaction (red) and a reaction with an inhibitor at its IC_{50} concentration (blue). The inhibition values determined at different end-points throughout the progress curve are shown in green. Initial velocities are represented by dotted lines.

4.1.1.4. ORDER OF REAGENT ADDITION

The order of addition of reactants and putative inhibitors is important to modulate the sensitivity of an assay for slow binding and irreversible inhibitors.

A preincubation (usually 5–10 min) of enzyme and test compound favors the finding of slow binding competitive inhibitors. If the substrate is added first, these inhibitors have a lower probability of being found.

In some cases, especially for multisubstrate reactions, the order of addition can be engineered to favor certain uncompetitive inhibitors. For instance, a mimetic of an amino acid that could act as an inhibitor of one aminoacyl-tRNA synthetase will exhibit a much higher inhibition if preincubated with enzyme and ATP before addition of the amino acid substrate.

4.1.2. Binding Assays

Although this section is focused on receptor binding, other binding reactions (protein-protein, protein-nucleic acid, etc.) are governed by similar laws, and so assays to monitor these interactions should follow the guidelines hereby suggested (for more details, *see* Chapters 2 and 3).

4.1.2.1. Ligand Concentration

The equation that describes binding of a ligand to a receptor, developed by Langmuir to describe adsorption of gas films to solid surfaces, is virtually identical to the Michaelis-Menten equation for enzyme kinetics:

$$BL = B_{max} \times L / (Kd + L)$$

where BL = bound ligand concentration (equivalent to v_0), B_{max} = maximum binding capacity (equivalent to V_{max}), L = total ligand concentration (equivalent to S) and Kd = equilibrium affinity constant also known as dissociation constant (equivalent to Km).

Therefore, all equations disclosed in **Subheading 4.1.1.1.**, can be directly translated to ligand-binding assays. For example, for competitive binders,

$$IC_{50} = (1 + L/Kd) \times Ki$$

Uncompetitive binders cannot be detected in binding assays; functional assays must be performed to detect this inhibitor class. Allosteric binders could be found if their binding modifies the receptor in a fashion that prevents ligand binding.

Typically, ligand concentration is set at the Kd concentration as an optimal way to attain a good signal (50% of binding sites occupied). This results in a good sensitivity for finding competitive binders.

4.1.2.2. Receptor Concentration

The same principles outlined for enzyme concentration in **Subheading 4.1.1.2.** apply to receptor concentration, or concentration of partners in other binding assays. In most cases, especially with membrane-bound receptors, the nominal concentration of receptor is not known. It can be determined by measuring the proportion of bound ligand at the Kd. In any case, linearity of response (binding) with respect to receptor (membrane) concentration should be assessed.

In traditional radiofiltration assays, it was recommended to set the membrane concentration so as to reach at most 10% of ligand bound at the Kd concentration, i.e., the concentration of receptor present should be below 1/5 of Kd *(13)*. Although this is appropriate to get accurate binding constants, it is not absolutely required to find competitive binders in a screening assay. Some formats (FP, SPA in certain cases) require a higher proportion of ligand bound to achieve acceptable statistics, and receptor concentrations close or above the Kd value have to be used.

Another variable to be considered in ligand-binding assays is nonspecific binding (NSB) of the labeled ligand. NSB increases linearly with membrane concentration. High NSB leads to unacceptable assay statistics, but this can often be improved with various buffer additives (*see* **Subheading 4.2.**).

4.1.2.3. Pre-incubation and Equilibrium

As discussed for enzymatic reactions, a preincubation of test compounds with the receptor would favor slow binders. After the preincubation step, the ligand is added and the binding reaction should be allowed to reach equilibrium in order to ensure a proper calculation of displacement by putative inhibitors. Running binding assays at equilibrium is convenient for HTS assays, since one does not have to carefully control the time between addition of ligand and assay readout as long as the equilibrium is stable.

4.1.3. Cell-Based Assays

The focus of the previous sections has been on cell-free systems. Cell-based assays offer different challenges in their set-up with many built-in factors that are out of the scientist's control. Nevertheless, some of the points discussed earlier apply to them, *mutatis mutandi*. A few general points to consider are:

- The response observed should be linear with respect to the number of cells;
- Pre-incubation of cells with compounds should be considered when applicable (e.g., assays in which a ligand is added); and
- Optimal incubation time should be selected in accordance to the rule of avoiding underestimation of inhibition or activation values (*see* **Subheading 4.1.1.3.**).

4.2. Assay Optimization

In vitro assays are performed in artificial environments in which the biological system studied could be unstable or exhibiting an activity below its potential. The requirements for stability are higher in HTS campaigns than in other areas of research. In HTS runs, diluted solutions of reagents are used throughout long periods of time (typically 4–12 h) and there is a need to keep both the variability low and the signal to background high. Additionally, several hundreds of thousands of samples are usually tested, and economics often dictates one to reduce the amount of reagents required. In this respect, miniaturization of assay volumes has been in continuous evolution, from tubes to 96-well plates to 384-well plates to 1536 and beyond. Many times, converting assays from low density to high-density formats is not straightforward. Thus, in order to find the best possible conditions for evaluating an HTS target, optimization of the assay should be accomplished as part of the development phase.

HTS libraries contain synthetic compounds or natural extracts that in most cases are dissolved in dimethyl sulfoxide (DMSO). The tolerance of the assay to DMSO should be considered. If significant decrease on activity/binding is observed at the standard solvent concentration—typically 0.5–1% (v/v) DMSO—lower concentrations may be required. In some cases the detrimental effect of solvent can be circumvented by the optimized assay conditions.

The stability of reagents should be tested using the same conditions intended for HTS runs, including solvent concentration, stock concentration of reagents, reservoirs, plates, etc. Sometimes signal is lost with time not because of degradation of one biological partner in the reaction but because of its adsorption to the plastics used (reservoir, tips, or plates) (**Fig. 4**).

The number of factors that can be tested in an optimization process is immense. Nevertheless, initial knowledge of the system (optimal pH, metal requirements, sensitivity to oxidation, etc.) can help to select the most appropriate ones. Factors to be considered can be grouped as follows:

- Buffer composition
- pH
- Temperature
- Ionic strength
- Osmolarity
- Monovalent ions (Na^+, K^+, Cl^-)
- Divalent cations (Mn^{2+}, Mg^{2+}, Ca^{2+}, Zn^{2+}, Cu^{2+}, Co^{2+})
- Reological modulators (glycerol, polyethyleneimine glycol [PEG])
- Polycations (heparin, dextran)
- Carrier-proteins (bovine serum albumin [BSA], casein)
- Chelating agents (ethylene diamine tetraacetic acid [EDTA], ethylene glyrol tetraacetic acid [EGTA])
- Blocking agents (polyethyleneimine [PEI], milk powder)
- Reducing agents (dithiothreitol [DTT], β-mercaptoethanol)
- Protease inhibitors (phenylmethylsulfonyl fluoride [PMSF], leupeptin)
- Detergents (Triton, Tween, CHAPS)

In addition, there are other factors that need to be specifically optimized for some techniques. For instance, SPA for receptor-binding assays can be performed with different types of beads, and the concentration of bead itself should be carefully selected according to the behavior of every receptor (Bmax, NSB, Kd, etc.). Cell-based assays are usually conducted in cell media of complex formulation. Factors to be considered in this case are mainly medium, supplier, selection, and concentration of extra protein (human serum albumin, BSA, gelatin, collagen). One also needs to take into account the possible physiological role of the factors chosen and also the cell's tolerance to them.

Besides analyzing the effect of factors individually, it is important to consider interactions between factors because synergies and antagonisms can commonly occur *(14)*. Full-factorial or partial factorial designs can be planned using several available statistical packages (e.g., JMP, Statistica, Design Expert). Experimental designs result in quite complex combinations as soon as more than four factors are tested. This task becomes rather complicated in high-density formats when taking into consideration that more reliable data are obtained if

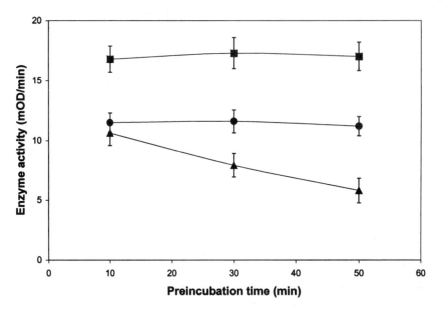

Fig. 4. Example of loss of signal in an enzymatic reaction related with adsorption of enzyme (or substrate) to plasticware. The data is from a real assay performed in our lab. Stability of reagents was initially measured using polypropylene tubes and 384-well polystyrene plates, without CHAPS (circles). Once HTS was started, using polypropylene reservoirs and polystyrene 384-well plates (triangles), a clear loss of signal was observed. Addition of 0.01% (w/v) CHAPS not only solved the problem but improved the enzyme activity (squares). Reactions were initiated at 10, 30, and 50 min after preparation of diluted stocks of reagents that remained at 4°C before addition to the reaction wells.

tests are performed randomly. Therefore, an automated solution is necessary because manually running an experiment of this complexity would be extremely difficult. A full package called AAO (automated assay optimization) has been recently launched by Beckman Coulter (Fullerton, CA) in collaboration with scientists from GlaxoSmithKline *(15)*. An example of the outcome of one assay recently improved in our lab using this methodology is shown in **Fig. 5**. The paper by Taylor et al. *(15)* describes examples of assay optimization through AAO for several type of targets and assay formats.

A typical optimization process starts with a partial factorial design including many factors (**ref. 20**). The most promising factors are then tested in a full-factorial experiment to analyze not only main effects but also two-factor interactions. These experiments are done with two levels per factor (very often one level is absence of the ingredient and the other is presence at a fairly typical concentration). Finally, titrations of the more beneficial factors are conducted in order to find optimal concentrations of every component.

Usually the focus of optimization is on activity (signal or signal to background), but statistical performance should also be taken into account when doing assay optimization. Though this is not feasible when many factors and levels are scrutinized without replicates, whenever possible duplicates or triplicates should be run and the resulting variability measured for every condition. Some buffer ingredients make a reproducible dispensement very difficult, and so should only be used if they are really beneficial (e.g., glycerol).

For some factors it is critical to run the HTS assay close to physiological conditions (e.g., pH) in order to avoid missing interesting leads for which the chemical structure or interaction with the target may change as a function of that factor.

4.3. Statistical Evaluation of HTS Assay Quality

The quality of a HTS assay must be determined according to its primary goal, i.e., to distinguish accurately hits from nonhits in a vast collection of samples.

In the initial evaluation of assay performance, several plates are filled with positive controls (signal; e.g., uninhibited enzyme reaction) and negative controls or blanks (background; e.g., substrate without enzyme). Choosing the right blank is sometimes not so obvious. In ligand-receptor binding assays, the blanks referred to as NSB controls are prepared traditionally by adding an excess of unlabeled (cold) ligand; the resulting displacement could be unreachable for some specific competitors that would not prevent NSB of the labeled ligand to membranes, or labware. A better blank could be prepared with membranes from the same cell line not expressing the receptor targeted. Though this is not always practical in the HTS context, it should be at least tested in the development of the assay, and compared with the NSB controls to which they should be, ideally, fairly close.

A careful analysis of these control plates allows identifying errors in liquid handling or sample processing. For instance, an assay with a long incubation typically produces plates with edge effects due to faster evaporation of the external wells even if lids are used, unless the plates are placed in a chamber with humidity control. Analysis of patterns (per row, per column, per quadrant) helps to identify systematic liquid-handling errors.

Obvious problems must be solved before evaluating the quality of the assay. After troubleshooting, random errors are still expected to happen due to instrument failure or defects in the labware used. They should be included in the subsequent analysis of performance (removing outliers is a misleading temptation equivalent to hiding the dirt under the carpet).

A

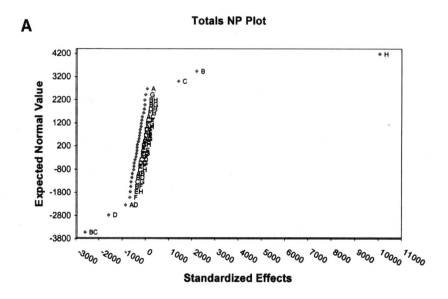

B

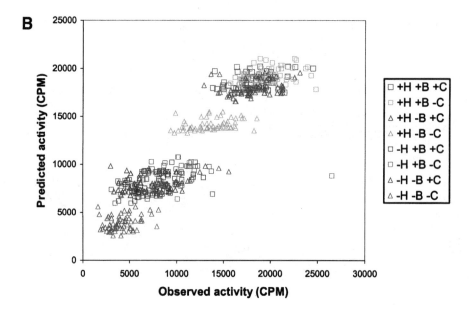

The analysis of performance can be accomplished by several means. Graphical analysis helps to identify systematic errors (e.g., **Fig. 6**). The statistical analysis of raw data involves the calculations of a number of parameters, starting with mean (M) and standard deviations (SD) for signal and background, and combinations of these as follows:

1. Signal to background

$$S/B = M_{signal} / M_{background}$$

   S/B provides an indication of the separation of positive and negative controls. It has to be reviewed in the context of the assay technique used. In our experience, a S/B of 3 is the minimal requirement for a robust assay, though some techniques less prone to variability allow for lower S/B ratios (e.g., FP). While assay variability is instrument dependent and can change from experiment to experiment, S/B is mainly assay-dependent and can be used early on to estimate the quality of an assay.

2. Specific signal or signal window

$$SW = M_{signal} - M_{background}$$

   SW gives another idea of the magnitude of the signal. It has to be reviewed in the context of the assay technique used. For instance, at least 1,000 CPM in a radiometric assay or 5 mOD/min in a continuous absorbance assay are required to avoid reproducibility problems in the subsequent HTS campaign.

Fig. 5. (Left) Example of optimization of a radiofiltration assay using Beckman Coulter's AAO program and a Biomek 2000 to perform the liquid handling. The target was to increase activity of this enzyme, aiming to improve assay quality and reduce costs. The initial partial factorial test included 20 factors, 8 of which were identified as positive. The test shown in this figure used these 8 factors and was designed as a 2-level full factorial experiment with duplicates. 512 samples were generated. (**A**) The probability plot resulting from the statistical analysis of experimental data showed three factors being positive (H, B, and C) although the interaction of B and C was negative. D showed significant negative effect, while the other four factors had statistically marginal or no effect. (**B**) Applying the statistical model, the correlation between observed and predicted values was very good. The presence of H = CHAPS 0.03 % (w/v) (+H red and orange, –H dark and light blue) is clearly positive. In the absence of B = 125 m*M* Bicine (+B squares, –B triangles) and C = 125 m*M* TAPS (+C red and dark blue, –C orange and light blue), the enzyme was less active. The original conditions yielded ca. 5,000 CPM vs ca. 25,000 CPM with the optimized buffer (backgrounds were ca. 100 CPM in all cases).

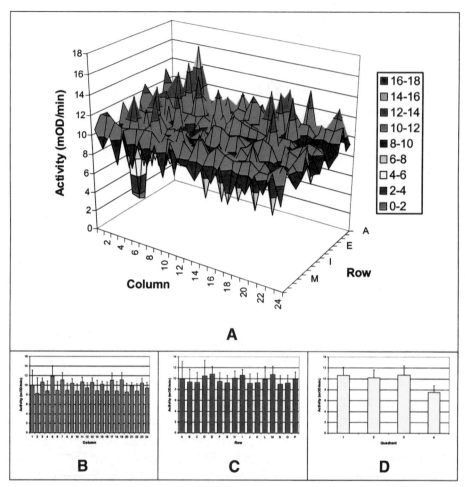

Fig. 6. Graphical analysis of a 384-well plate of positive controls of an enzymatic reaction monitored by absorbance (continuous read-out). The plate was filled using a pipettor equipped with a 96-well head and indexing capability. (**A**) Three-dimensional plot of the whole plate showing that four wells (I1, I2, J1, and J2) had a dispensement problem. The corresponding tip may have been loose or clogged. Analysis by columns (**B**), rows (**C**), and quadrants (**D**) reveals that the 4th quadrant was receiving less reagent.

3. Signal to noise

$$S/N = (M_{signal} - M_{background}) / SD_{background}$$

This classic expression of S/N provides an incomplete combination of signal window and variability. Its original purpose was to assess the separation between signal and background in a radio signal *(16)*. It should not be used to evaluate performance of HTS assays.

Another parameter referred to as S/N by some authors is:

$$S/N = (M_{signal} \ 2 \ M_{background}) \ / \ \sqrt{(SD_{signal})^2 + (SD_{background})^2}$$

This second expression provides a complete picture of the performance of a HTS assay. Typically, assays with values of S/N greater than 10 are considered acceptable.

4. Coefficient of variation of signal and background

$$CV = 100 \times SD/M \ (\%)$$

A relative measure of variability, it provides a good indication of variability for the signal. For backgrounds it is less useful, as values close to 0 for the mean distort the CV. Variability is a function of the assay stability and precision of liquid handling and detection instruments.

5. Z' factor

$$Z' = 1 - 3 \times (SD_{signal} + SD_{background}) \ / \ |M_{signal} - M_{background}|$$

Since its publication in 1999 *(16)* the Z' factor has been widely accepted by the HTS community as a very useful way of assessing the statistical performance of an assay. Z' is an elegant combination of signal window and variability, the main parameters used in the evaluation of assay quality. The relationship between Z' factor and S/B is not obvious from its definition but can be easily derived as:

$$Z' = 1 - 0.03 \times (|S/B| \times CV_{signal} + CV_{background}) \ / \ (|S/B| - 1)$$

The value of Z' factor is a relative indication of the separation of the signal and background populations. It is assumed that there is a normal distribution for these populations, as is the case if the variability is due to random errors.

Z' factor is a dimensionless parameter that ranges from 1 (infinite separation) to < 0. Signal and background populations start to overlap when Z' = 0. In our lab, the acceptance criteria for an assay is Z' > 0.4, equivalent to having a S/B of 3 and a CV of 10%. Higher S/B ratios allow for higher variability, but as a rule, the CV_{signal} must be below 20%. Low variability allows for a lower S/B, but a minimum of 2 is usually required provided that CV_{signal} is rarely below 5%. **Figure 7** shows Z' at work in 3 different scenarios. Full analysis of the corresponding data is collected in **Table 3**.

Z' should be evaluated during assay development and validation, and also throughout HTS campaigns on a per plate basis to assess the quality of dispensement and reject data from plates with errors.

4.4. Assay Validation

Once an assay optimized to find compounds of interest passes its quality control with a Z' greater than 0.4 (or whatever is the applied acceptance criteria),

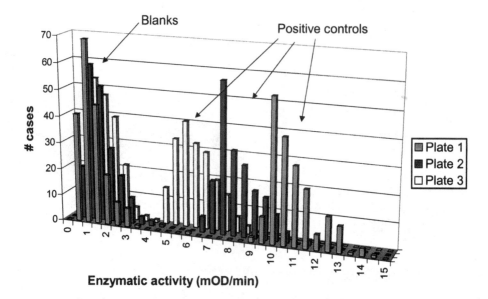

Fig. 7. Distribution of activity values (bins of 0.5 mOD/min) for three 384-well plates half-filled with blanks and half-filled with positive controls of an enzymatic reaction monitored by absorbance (continuous read-out). Z' factors were 0.59 for plate 1, 0.42 for plate 2, and 0.10 for plate 3. A complete analysis of performance is shown in **Table 3**.

Table 3
Statistical Analysis of Data from the Three Plates Described in Fig. 7

Parameter	Plate 1	Plate 2	Plate 3
M_{signal} (mOD/min)	10.09	7.77	5.84
SD_{signal} (mOD/min)	0.84	0.81	0.96
$M_{background}$ (mOD/min)	0.30	0.69	0.74
$SD_{background}$ (mOD/min)	0.51	0.57	0.57
S/B	34	11	8
SW (mOD/min)	9.80	7.08	5.09
S/N[a]	19	12	9
S/N[b]	10.0	7.1	4.6
CV_{signal} (%)	8%	10%	16%
$CV_{background}$ (%)	173%	82%	77%
Z' factor	0.59	0.42	0.10

[a]$S/N = (M_{signal} - M_{background}) / SD_{background}$

[b]$S/N = (M_{signal} - M_{background}) / \sqrt{(SD_{signal})^2 + (SD_{background})^2}$

a final step must be done before starting a HTS campaign. The step referred to here as assay validation consists of testing a representative sample of the screening collection in the same way HTS plates will be treated; i.e., on the same robotic system using protocols identical to the HTS run. The purposes of this study are to:

1. Obtain field data on assay performance,
2. Estimate the hit rate and determination of optimal sample concentration,
3. Assess interferences from screening samples, and
4. Evaluate the reproducibility of results obtained in a production environment

The size of the pilot collection can be as small as 1% of the total collection. Its usefulness to predict hit rates and interferences increases with its size. On the other hand, too many plates worth of work and reagents can be lost if any major problem is found in this step, as often happens. Therefore, it is not advisable to go beyond a 5% representation of the collection.

With a randomized sample of 1% of a collection of 50,000 compounds, a hit rate of 1% can be estimated with a SD of 0.5%. For a 5% rate, the estimation's SD would be 1% (approximate figures calculated as described in *17*).

Irrespective of the size of the pilot collection, at least 10–20 plates should be run to test the HTS system in real action. Duplicates of the same samples run in independent experiments provide a way to evaluate the reproducibility of results (**Fig. 8**).

A dramatic example of how the test of a pilot collection helps to detect interferences is shown in **Fig. 9**. This target had been tested for and found to be slightly unstable at room temperature (**Fig. 9B**, without BSA). Nevertheless, the effect of 352 mixtures of compounds was tested and an extremely high hit rate was observed (45% of the mixtures inhibited the enzyme activity greater than 70%). The problem was solved by stabilization of the system using BSA 0.05%. Similar effects have been observed in several other targets.

4.5. Summary

HTS is at the core of the drug-discovery process, and so it is critical to design and implement HTS assays in a comprehensive fashion involving scientists from the disciplines of biology, chemistry, engineering, and informatics. This requires careful analysis of many variables, starting with the choice of assay target and ending with the discovery of lead compounds. At every step in this process, there are decisions to be made that can greatly impact the outcome of the HTS effort, to the point of making it a success or a failure. Although specific guidelines can be established to ensure that the screening assay reaches an acceptable level of quality, many choices require pragmatism and the ability to compromise opposing forces.

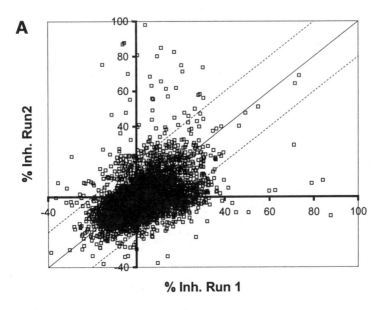

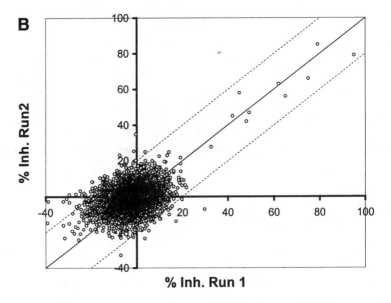

Fig. 8. Comparison of duplicates from validation for two HTS assays. **(A)** This enzymatic assay showed a significant number of mismatched results between duplicate runs of the same 4,000 samples. Two actions should be taken in a case like this: liquid handling errors have to be avoided, and the assay quality must be improved. **(B)** The data corresponds to a ligand-binding assay that showed a good reproducibility.

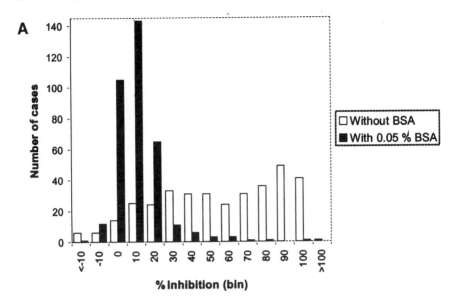

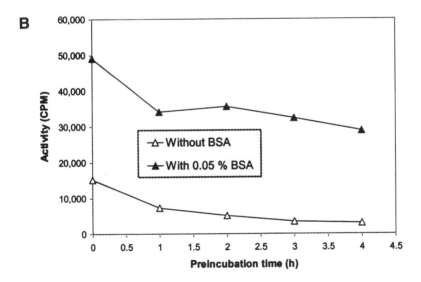

Fig. 9. (A) Distribution of inhibition values (10% bins) in the validation of a HTS assay of an enzyme tested with and without 0.05% (w/v) BSA. The samples were 352 representative mixtures of compounds (11 components at 9.1 μM each). (B) It was shown that the stability and activity of the enzyme was greatly improved in the presence of BSA.

Acknowledgments

The authors would like to thank Glenn Hofmann, Christina Schulz, Paul Taylor, and Walt deWolf for kindly providing unpublished data. We are grateful to them, Brian Bond, Fran Stewart, Andy Pope, and other colleagues at GlaxoSmithKline for their help to shape the screening process hereby described. Critical review of this chapter by Paul Taylor is also acknowledged.

References

1. Stadel, J. M., Wilson, S., and Bergsma, D. J. (1997) Orphan G protein-coupled receptors: a neglected opportunity for pioneer drug discovery. *Trends Pharmacol. Sci.* **18,** 430–437.
2. Cascieri, M. A., and Springer, M. S. (2000) The chemokine/chemokine-receptor family: potential and progress for therapeutic intervention. *Curr. Opin. Chem. Biol.* **4,** 420–427.
3. Miller, W. H., Alberts, D. P., Bhatnagar, P. K., et al. (2000) Discovery of orally active nonpeptide vitronectin receptor antagonists based on a 2-benzazepine Gly-Asp mimetic. *J. Med. Chem.* **43,** 22–26.
4. Gonzalez, J. E., Oades, K., Leychkis, Y., Harootunian, A., and Negulescu, P. A. (1999) Cell-based assays and instrumentation for screening ion-channel targets. *Drug Discov. Today* **4,** 431–439.
5. Schroeder, K. S., and Neagle, B. D. (1996) FLIPR: a new instrument for accurate, high throughput optical screening. *J. Biomol. Screen.* **1,** 75–80.
6. Hertzberg, R. P., and Pope, A. J. (2000) High throughput screening: new technology for the 21st century. *Curr. Opin. Chem. Biol.* **4,** 45–451.
7. Pope, A. J., Haupts, U., and Moore, K. J. (1999) Homogeneous fluorescence readouts for miniaturized high-throughput screening: theory and practice. *Drug Discov. Today* **4,** 350–362.
8. Ullman, D., Busch, M., and Mander, T. (1999) Fluorescence correlation spectroscopy-based screening technology. *J. Pharm. Technol.* **99,** 30–40.
9. Cheng, Y. C., and Prussof, W. (1973) Relationship between the inhibition constant (Ki) and the concentration of inhibitor which causes 50 per cent inhibition (I50) of an enzymatic reaction. *Biochem. Pharmacol.* **22,** 3099–3108.
10. Bush, K. (1983) Screening and characterization of enzyme inhibitors as drug candidates. *Drug Metab. Rev.* **14,** 689–708.
11. Macarron, R., Mensah, L., Cid, C., et al. (2000) A homogeneous method to measure aminoacyl-tRNA synthetase aminoacylation activity using scintillation proximity assay technology. *Anal. Biochem.* **284,** 183–190.
12. Tipton, K. F. (1980) Kinetics and enzyme inhibition studies, in Enzyme Inhibitors as Drugs (Sandler, M., ed.) University Park Press, Baltimore, MD.
13. Burt, D. (1986) Receptor binding methodology and analysis, in *Receptor Binding in Drug Research* (O'Brien, R. A., ed.) Marcel Dekker, NY, pp. 4–29.
14. Lutz, M.W., Menius, J.A., et al. (1996) Experimental design for high-throughput screening. *Drug Discov. Today* **1,** 277–286.

15. Taylor, P., Stewart, F., et al (2000) Automated assay optimization with integrated statistics and smart robotics. *J. Biomol. Screen.* **5,** 213–225.

16. Zhang, J. H., Chung, T. D. Y., and Oldenburg, K. R. (1999) A simple statistical parameter for use in evaluation and validation of high throughput screening assays. *J. Biomol. Screen.* **4,** 67–73.

17. Barnett, V. (1974) *Elements of sampling theory* English Universities Press, London, pp. 42–46.

2

Configuring Radioligand Receptor Binding Assays for HTS Using Scintillation Proximity Assay Technology

John W. Carpenter, Carmen Laethem, Frederick R. Hubbard, Thomas K. Eckols, Melvyn Baez, Don McClure, David L. G. Nelson, and Paul A. Johnston

1. Introduction

Rapid progress in the fields of genomics, proteomics, and molecular biology has both increased the numbers of potential drug targets, and facilitated development of assays to screen these targets *(1–5)*. In parallel with these changes, developments in robotics and combinatorial chemical synthesis have driven the production of very large numbers of compounds with potential for pharmacological activity *(1–5)*. The need to screen these large libraries of drug candidates against multiple new targets has stimulated improvements in technology, instrumentation, and automation that have revolutionized the field of drug discovery, and evolved into the field of high throughput screening (HTS) *(1,5–9)*. Radioligand binding assays have historically been the mainstay of drug discovery and drug development *(6–8)*. In the era of HTS, incorporation of scintillation-proximity technology together with improved automation and radiometric-counting instrumentation have served to maintain radioligand receptor-binding as one of the premier tools of drug discovery *(1,5,8,9)*. Radioligand binding assays are extremely versatile, easy to perform, can be automated to provide very high throughput *(10–12)*. The quality of the data allows the determination of drug affinity, allosteric interactions, the existence of receptor subtypes, and estimates of receptor numbers *(10–12)*. This chapter provides an overview of radioligand receptor-binding assays and discusses some of the issues associated with the conversion of traditional filtration assays

From: *Methods in Molecular Biology, vol. 190: High Throughput Screening: Methods and Protocols*
Edited by: W. P. Janzen © Humana Press Inc., Totowa, NJ

to a homogeneous scintillating proximity assay (SPA) format that is more compatible with automation and HTS.

1.1. Basic Radioligand-Binding Theory

The classical definition of a receptor involves a functional response, and while receptor binding should be saturable, reversible, and stereo-selective, functional activity is not measured in binding experiments (10–12). Despite recent developments in nonradioactive techniques like fluorescence polarization (13,14), radioligand-receptor binding is the most commonly used technique for the biochemical identification and pharmacological characterization of receptors in drug discovery (10–12). There are a number of excellent reviews that provide an overview of the theory and methodology of traditional radioligand receptor-binding assays, together with a discussion of the potential problems and artifacts associated with the various formats available (10–12,15–18). SPA radioligand receptor binding assays share the same issues as more traditional formats; choice of radioligand, selection of receptor preparation, optimization of assay conditions, and appropriate analysis of the data (1,8–12).

There are two major categories of radioligand binding studies: kinetic studies and equilibrium studies (10–12). Kinetic binding experiments typically define the time-course of ligand association and dissociation with the receptor, and are generally used to optimize binding conditions and demonstrate the reversibility of the ligand-receptor interactions (10–12). For drug-discovery purposes, saturation and competition (displacement) binding experiments are the two types of equilibrium (steady-state) binding studies most commonly utilized to estimate the classical binding parameters; the dissociation constant (K_d), the binding capacity (B_{max}), and the affinity (K_i) of a competing drug for the receptor ligand (10–12). Specific binding is the proportion of total binding of a radioligand to a receptor preparation that can be displaced by an unlabeled compound known to bind to the receptor of interest (10–12). Competition for receptor-binding sites might involve the same unlabeled chemical species as the radioligand (homologous displacement), or a different chemical species (heterologous displacement) (10–12). Nonspecific binding includes binding of the radioligand to glass-fiber filters, adsorption to the tissue, and dissolution in the membrane lipids (10–12). To reduce the chances of the unlabeled ligand displacing radioligand from saturable nonreceptor sites such as uptake carriers or enzymes, it is generally recommended that the displacing ligand should be structurally dissimilar from the radioligand. Operationally, nonspecific binding is defined as the amount of radioligand bound in the presence of an appropriate excess of unlabeled drug. An assay is considered barely adequate if 50% of the total binding is specific; 70% is good and 90% is excellent (10–12).

1.2. Filtration-Format Radioligand Binding

The basic outline of most radioligand binding assays is very similar; a preparation containing the receptor is incubated with a radioligand for a period of time, the bound ligand is separated from the free ligand, and the amount of radioligand bound is quantified by liquid-scintillation counting *(10–12)*. It is important to prevent significant dissociation of the receptor-radioligand during separation, a problem typically addressed by performing the separation as rapidly as possible, or at reduced temperature to slow the rate of dissociation *(10–12,15–18)*. Although centrifugation, dialysis, and gel filtration are options, the separation technique most widely used with membrane preparations and whole cells is filtration, either on a vacuum manifold or by a cell harvester *(10–12,15–18)*. The bound ligand is retained on glass-fiber filters, and the free ligand passes through. After the initial filtration, filters are rinsed extensively with assay buffer to reduce the level of nonspecific binding. Filters may also be prerinsed or presoaked with solutions such as 0.1% polyethylenimine to decrease nonspecific binding *(10–12)*. Characteristically, nonspecific binding attains steady-state more rapidly than specific binding, and increases linearly with the radioligand concentration rather than reaching saturation.

The relative ease of radioligand-binding assays together with the availability of radioligands for many different receptor types and the variety of receptor preparations that can be attained have all contributed to the popularity of the technique *(5–12)*. However, the physical separation of bound from free radioligand involving reagent transfer, filtration, and multiple wash steps, is a time consuming and relatively labor-intensive process that can significantly limit throughput in HTS. Filtration-binding assays also expose personnel to the hazards of manipulating radioactive solutions, and generate a significant volume of radioactive waste that is costly to dispose of *(1,8,9)*. In recent years, the development of the Multiscreen® Assay System (Millipore) of micotiter filter plates, the MAP® filter plate aspirator (Titertek), and photomultiplier tube (PMT) microplate liquid-scintillation counters (Wallac Microbeta®, & Packard Topcount®) have significantly improved the ability to automate filtration-binding assays for HTS *(6,19,20)*. However filtration screens generate more radioactive waste and are sufficiently labor-intensive that throughput is limited. The demands of HTS make other screening formats more desirable.

1.3. Scintillation Proximity Radioligand Binding Format

SPA technology is a radioisotopic homogeneous-assay system that requires no separation step and allows the design of high-throughput receptor-binding assays that rely on pipetting in a "mix and measure" format *(1,8,9)*. SPA involves the use of fluoromicrosphere beads containing scintillant that are coated with acceptor molecules to capture biologically active molecules such as receptors, which can in turn bind radioactive ligands *(1,8,9)*. When the radioligand binds to a receptor coupled to the bead, the radioisotope is brought in close proximity to the scintillant and effective energy transfer from the beta-particle will take place, resulting in the emission of light *(1,8,9)*. No light is detected from unbound radioligand in free solution because the beta-particle released has a minimum path length of decay that is too distant from the scintillant in the bead, and the energy is dissipated in the assay buffer *(1,8,9)*. The homogeneous receptor binding format provides the ability to measure weak interactions without disturbing the equilibrium with a separation step, and makes it possible to monitor the rate of association or dissociation of a radioligand from its receptor *(1,8,9)*.

1.4. Conversion of a Filtration Radioligand Binding Assay to an SPA Format

While radioligand-binding assays may be directly configured in SPA format for HTS, it is preferable to first develop a filtration assay. The more traditional filtration assay may be used to compare and validate the SPA format, and many of the critical experimental variables defined in the filtration assay may be directly transferable to the SPA format, including; selection of radioligand, choice of receptor preparation, buffer composition, pH, temperature, and reaction time.

1.5. Selection of Radioligand

The important characteristics to be considered for the selection of the radioligand include the radioisotope, the extent of nonspecific binding, the selectivity and affinity for the receptor, and whether the radioligand is an agonist or an antagonist *(10–12)*. The radioligand must be soluble and stable in the incubation medium. Each radioligand has a unique pharmacological profile and the one utilized should bind selectively to the receptor type, or subtypes, of interest under the assay conditions used. Usually, high-affinity ligands are preferred because a lower concentration of radioligand can be used in the assay, resulting in lower levels of nonspecific binding, and a slower rate of dissociation *(10–12)*. Agonists may label only a subset of the total receptor population (high affinity state for G-protein coupled receptors [GPCR's]), whereas antagonists generally label all available receptors *(10–12)*.

Although ^{33}P and ^{35}S are occasionally used, ^{3}H and ^{125}I are the isotopes most commonly used to label ligands for binding assays *(10–12)*. It is important that the radioligand should have sufficient specific activity to allow accurate detection of low levels of binding *(10–12)*. The selection of radioisotope is especially critical for SPA, because the basis of the proximity effect is that an emitted β particle will only travel a limited distance in an aqueous environment, and that path length is dependent on the energy of the emitted particle *(1,8,9)*. In order for the radioactive disintegration to be detected, the β particle must interact with the scintillant in the bead, resulting in energy transfer and emission of light. Electrons from ^{3}H have a range of energies leading to an average path length of 1.5 µm, and the two monoenergetic internal-conversion electrons emitted by ^{125}I have path lengths of 1 µm and 17.5 µm, respectively. ^{3}H and ^{125}I are ideally suited to SPA in that only bound ligands brought in close proximity to the scintillant will generate a signal. In contrast, ^{14}C, ^{35}S, and ^{33}P have path lengths with mean ranges of 58, 66, and 126 µm, respectively, that are less suited to the proximity principle due to the higher signals produced by unbound radioactive ligand *(1,8,9)*.

1.6. Selection of Receptor Preparation

Radioligand binding is an extremely versatile technique that can be applied to a wide variety of receptor preparations including purified and solubilized receptors, membrane preparations, whole cells, and tissue slices *(10–12)*. Membrane preparations are the most widely utilized receptor source, but access to the receptor of interest, especially human receptors, remains a critical issue. The advent of molecular- and cell-biology techniques to clone and express human receptors have been enabling technologies for HTS that have provided access to cell lines with high receptor-expression levels *(2,3,5)*. Stable cell lines can be expanded in cell culture to high density and crude membrane fractions may be easily generated by the differential centrifugation of cells homogenized in a hypotonic buffer *(8)* (*see* below). A more pragmatic solution may be to purchase the receptor sample of interest from a number of commercial sources that provide a quality controlled and validated preparation that comes unencumbered with intellectual property issues. Although these reagents may appear expensive, this may be offset by reduced in house development costs.

1.7. Selection of SPA Bead

SPA beads are available in two types, Yttrium silicate (Ysi) or Polyvinyltoluene (PVT). PVT beads containing diphenylanthracine (DPA) have an average diameter of 5 µm, a density of 1.05 g/cm^3 and a typical counting efficiency of 40% compared to liquid scintillation counting. Ysi beads have scintillant properties by virtue of cerium ions within the crystal lattice, have an average diameter of 2.5 µm, a density of ~4.0 g/cm^3 and a typical counting efficiency of 60% compared to liquid-scintillation counting. Although Ysi is one of the most efficient solid scintillators known and provides a higher output than PVT beads in SPA assays, PVT beads are less dense and more compatible with automation. A variety of coupling molecules are available for binding receptor preparations to the surface of SPA beads. These include wheat germ agglutinin (WGA), streptavidin, poly-L-lysine, protein A, glutathione, copper his-tag, antirabbit, antimouse, antisheep, and antiguinea pig antibodies. The binding capacity of the beads for the receptor preparation and the level of nonspecific interaction with the radioligand, are both important criteria to be evaluated before selection of bead type and coupling molecule.

1.8. Buffer Composition

Radioligand binding to membrane preparations can often be achieved in relatively simple buffer solutions such as HEPES (10–20 mM), Tris-HCl (10–170 mM), or phosphate buffers (30 mM), generally in the physiological range of pH 7.0 to 8.0 *(10–12)*. Ionic composition may be important, and cations such as Na^+, Mg^{2+} and Ca^{2+} are frequently included in buffers to either enhance specific binding, or inhibit nonspecific binding *(10–12)*. GTP is sometimes included in the buffers for GPCR binding assays because it can modulate agonist affinity for the receptor and convert a complex inhibition curve (biphasic) to a simple (single-site) inhibition curve *(10)*. It is important that the radioligand and receptor should be stable throughout the incubation period. It is not uncommon to include antioxidants such as ascorbic acid, or enzyme inhibitors such as pargyline, a monoamine oxidase inhibitor, in the assay buffer to control chemical and enzymatic stability *(10–12)*. Similarly, a variety of protease inhibitors and chelating agents such as ethyleneglycoltetraacetic acid (EGTA) or ethylenediamine tetraacetic acid (EDTA) may be included to preserve receptors and ligands from proteolytic degradation *(10–12)*. Typically, the conversion of a filtration binding assay to an SPA format does not require a change in the assay buffer *(8)*.

2. Materials

2.1. Cell Culture

1. AV12 cells (Syrian Hamster fibroblasts, ATCC # CRL 9595).
2. Methotrexate or hygromycin.

2.2. Membrane Preparation

1. 50 mM Tris-HCl, pH 7.4.
2. Bicinchoninic acid (BCA) kit; Micro BCA™ Protein Assay Reagent (Pierce, Rockford, IL).

2.3. Filtration Format Receptor Binding Assay

1. Binding assay buffer: 50 mM Tris-HCl, 0.5 mM EDTA, 10 mM $MgSO_4$, 0.1%. Ascorbic acid, 10 μM Pargyline, pH 7.75 at 25°C.

2. 5-Hydroxy(^{3}H)tryptamine trifluoroacetate (Code TRK1006 Amersham, Piscataway, NJ) at a final concentration of 5 nM per well.
3. Beta Plate scintillation counter (Perkin Elmer Wallac Inc., Gaithersburg, MD).

2.4. SPA Format Receptor Binding Assay

1. Binding Assay Buffer: 50 mM Tris-HCl, 0.5 mM EDTA, 10 mM MgSO$_4$, 0.1% Ascorbic Acid, 10 μM Pargyline, pH 7.75 at 25°C).
2. 5-Hydroxy(^{3}H)tryptamine trifluoroacetate (Code TRK1006 Amersham) at a final concentration of 5 nM/well.
3. Wheat-germ agglutinin (WGA) SPA beads were obtained from Amersham Pharmacia Biotech.
4. Microbeta Scintillation Counter (Perkin Elmer Wallac).

2.5. Automation used for High Throughput SPA Assay

1. Multidrop (TiterTek Instruments, Huntsville, AL).
2. Megaflex (Tecan US, Durham, NC).
3. SLT Dispenser (Tecan US).
4. ORCA arm robotic system (Beckman Coulter, Fullerton, CA).
5. Microbeta Scintillation Counter (Perkin Elmer Wallac).

3. Methods

3.1. Cell Culture

The generation of AV12 cells stably transfected with the eukaryotic expression vector phd containing the coding region for the human 5HT$_{2C}$ receptor was described previously *(3)*. AV12 cell lines were grown in suspension with selection for resistance to methotrexate or hygromycin *(3)*.

3.2. Membrane Preparation

The preparation of membranes has been described previously *(8)*. Briefly:

1. Suspension cells are grown in a stirred 30-L fermenter (37°C, 5% CO$_2$) to a cell density of $2 - 3 \times 10^6$ cells/mL, and 15 L are harvested on a daily basis by centrifugation, washed in phosphate-buffered saline (PBS), and stored as frozen cell pastes at $- 80$°C.
2. To loosen the frozen cell paste, 30 mL of 50 mM Tris-HCl, pH 7.4, at ambient temperature are added to 7.5 grams of pellet.
3. The cell slurry is homogenized on ice in a 55-mL glass/teflon dounce, transferred to a 250-mL conical tube that is then filled to the neck with buffer, mixed, and centrifuged in a table top centrifuge at 200g (1060 RPM, GH-3.7 rotor) at 4°C for 15 min.
4. The supernatant is collected and saved on ice.
5. The pellet is resuspended and subjected to the homogenization and centrifugation procedure just described.

6. The 200*g* supernatant is again collected and combined with the first supernatant stored on ice.
7. The combined supernatants are then centrifuged at 14,250 rpm in a Sorvall RC5 centrifuge (GSA SLA-1500 rotor) for 50 min at 4°C.
8. The supernatant is gently removed and discarded, and the remaining membrane pellet is resuspended using the dounce homogenizer.
9. The membrane protein concentration is determined (BCA kit) and aliquots of the membrane preparation are quick frozen in liquid nitrogen and stored at –80°C. The average yield is 1.2% of starting weight.

3.3. Filtration-Format Receptor-Binding Assay

1. Fifty microliter of compound, unlabeled 5HT or binding buffer are added to each well of a 96-well microtiter plate, followed by 50 μL of 20 nM ^{3}H-5HT, and 100 μL (20 μg) of the 5HT$_{2C}$ membrane preparation.
2. Plates are sealed, placed on an orbital shaker for 2 min at setting 6, and then incubated for 30 min at 37°C.
3. The film is removed, 50 μL of 25% TCA is added to terminate the reaction, and the well contents are aspirated and transferred to a glass-fiber filter mat with a TomTec® cell harvester. After three wash cycles with ice-cold binding buffer, the filter mats are removed and dried in the microwave oven for 1 min.
4. Filter mats are then placed in a plastic bag, scintillation fluid is added, the fluid is spread out to cover the whole filter and air bubbles are removed with a rolling pin. The plastic bag is sealed with a heat-seal apparatus, mounted in a rack, and counted in a Beta Plate counter.

3.4. SPA-Format Receptor-Binding Assay

1. Twenty microliter of compound, unlabeled 5-HT, or assay buffer is added to each well of a 96-well microtiter plate.
2. Fifty microliter of 15-nM [^{3}H]-5HT ligand is then added to the wells followed by 80 μL of 5HT$_{2C}$ membranes (20 μg; *see* **Notes 5** and **6**) and the plates are shaken for 1 min.
3. After a 30-min incubation at room temperature, 0.5 mg of WGA-SPA beads are added (*see* **Notes 3**, **4**, and **7**), plates are mixed by shaking every 30 min for 2 h and then counted in a MicroBeta counter (*see* **Notes 9** and **19**).

3.5. Automation Used for High Throughput SPA Assay

1. The assay is as described in **Subheading 3.4.**
2. Compounds delivered as dimethyl sulfoxide (DMSO) stocks in 96-well plates are diluted in binding buffer added by Multidrop.
3. Diluted compounds and controls are transferred and added to assay plates using a Megaflex.
4. Membranes and radioligands are added to assay plates with an SLT Dispenser.
5. WGA-SPA beads are kept in suspension in binding buffer by a magnetic stir bar and added to assay plates by a Megaflex.

6. Plates are shaken on a Hotel Shaker and an ORCA arm robotic system is used to move plates between and load them into workstations.
7. Plates are counted in a Wallac Microbeta (6-Detector counter).

4. Notes

1. We will now describe the conversion of a radioligand receptor binding assay from a filtration to a SPA format, compatible with HTS. To illustrate this process and provide an example for discussion, we have selected a member of the 5-hydroxytryptamine (5-HT, Serotonin) receptor family that have been implicated in a variety of pathological conditions including anxiety, depression, aggressiveness, obsessive-compulsive behavior, schizophrenia, eating disorders, and alcoholism *(2,3,8)*. With the exception of 5-HT$_3$, which is a ligand gated ion channel, 5-HT receptors belong to the superfamily of GPCRs. There are seven receptor subtypes 5-HT$_{1-7}$, based on radioligand-binding properties, signal transduction mechanisms, and deduced amino acid sequences *(2,3,8)*.

4.1. Filtration Format Assay

2. A filtration format radioligand-binding assay (described in **Subheading 3.3.**), using ^{3}H-5HT as the ligand and membranes prepared from AV12 cells expressing the human 5HT$_{2C}$ receptor, had been developed and is to be converted to SPA format for HTS (**Fig. 1**). ^{3}H-5HT exhibited saturation binding to 20 µg of 5-HT$_{2C}$ membranes in the filtration assay, and the K$_d$ of 4.5 nM for 5-HT binding is consistent with published data *(2,3,8)*. At 3 nM ^{3}H-5HT, specific binding is 82% of the total binding observed, indicating a very good assay.

4.2. Optimization of SPA-Format Assay

3. Based on previous experience *(8)*, WGA-PVT beads were selected for an initial evaluation of the SPA format (**Fig. 2**).
4. Three variations on the SPA format are possible; membranes may be precoupled to the beads prior to the addition of ligand, all components of the assay can be added together at T$_0$, or beads can be added after the receptors and ligand have been incubated together. There are advantages and disadvantages to each assay format, depending on the ligand and receptor preparation of interest. Although it adds an extra step, one possible advantage of the precoupled format is that excess uncoupled membranes can be removed prior to the assay thereby ensuring that only binding sites coupled to beads are available. We selected the delayed format of bead addition for the example we will discuss.
5. Five nanomolar [^{3}H]-5HT ligand and the indicated amounts of 5HT$_{2C}$ membranes were added to wells as described in **Subheading 3.4.** Total binding increased with the amount of 5HT$_{2C}$ membranes added in a dose dependent manner up to ~20 µg/well, then reached a plateau such that no significant increase in signal was achieved with addition of more membranes. The data are consistent with saturation of the binding capacity of the WGA-SPA beads at 20–30 µg of membrane protein.

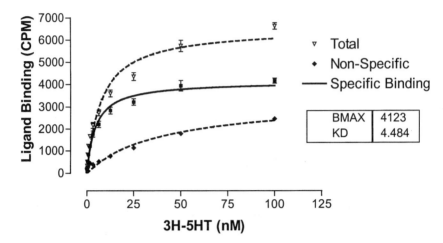

Fig. 1. Saturation binding of ^{3}H-5HT to 5-HT$_{2C}$ membranes filtration format. Compound, unlabeled 5-HT or binding buffer were incubated for 30 min at 37°C with the indicated amounts of ^{3}H-5HT and 20 µg of 5HT$_{2C}$ membranes. The contents of the wells were transferred onto a filter mat and washed using a TomTec® cell harvester, and filters were counted in a Beta Plate counter as described in Materials and Methods. Each point represents the mean +/– SDM of quadruplicate determinations.

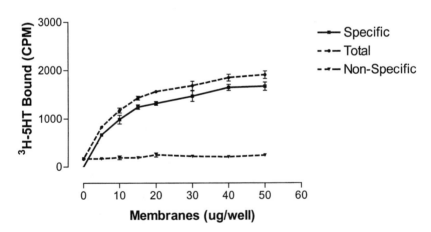

Fig. 2. Specific ^{3}H-5HT binding to 5HT$_{2C}$ membranes coupled to WGA-PVT SPA beads. Unlabeled 5-HT (10 µ*M*), assay buffer , [^{3}H]-5-HT ligand and the indicated amounts of 5HT$_{2C}$ membranes were incubated for 30 min at room temperature. One milligram of WGA-PVT SPA beads were added, plates were mixed by shaking every 30 min for 2 h and then counted in a MicroBeta (Wallac) counter as described in Materials and Methods. Each point represents the mean +/– SDM of quadruplicate determinations.

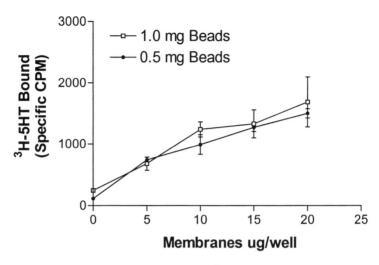

Fig. 3. Effect of bead amount on the specific ^{3}H-5HT binding to 5HT$_{2C}$ Membranes Coupled to WGA-PVT SPA Beads. Unlabeled 5-HT (10 μM), assay buffer, 5 nM [^{3}H]-5-HT ligand and the indicated amounts of 5HT$_{2C}$ membranes, were incubated for 30 min at room temperature. Either 0.5 mg or 1.0 mg of WGA-PVT SPA beads were added, plates were mixed by shaking every 30 min for 2 h and then counted in a MicroBeta (Wallac) counter as described in Materials and Methods. Each point represents the mean +/– SDM of quadruplicate determinations.

6. For all of the membrane concentrations tested, specific binding exceeded 80% of the total binding observed.

7. Since SPA beads are one of the more expensive components of the assay, we also performed a membrane-titration experiment with half the amount of beads (**Fig. 3**), and found that in the range tested, 0.5 mg was as effective as 1.0 mg of beads.

8. On the basis of these data, 20 μg/well of membranes and 0.5 mg/well of WGA-PVT beads were selected for an evaluation of saturation binding (**Fig. 4**). ^{3}H-5HT exhibits saturation binding to 20 μg of 5-HT$_{2C}$ membranes in the SPA assay, and the K_d of 3.0 nM for 5-HT binding is consistent with both the filtration assay (**Fig. 1**) and published data *(2,3,8)*. At 2.5 nM ^{3}H-5HT, specific binding was 94.6% of the total binding observed, indicating a very good assay.

9. Consistent with the lower counting efficiency of the SPA PVT-beads, the B$_{max}$ for the SPA format was 3279 CPMs compared to 4123 CPMs for the filtration assay.

10. To further validate the assay format we analyzed four known serotonergic compounds and unlabeled 5-HT in heterologous and homologous displacement binding assays (**Fig. 5**). The rank potency of the compounds tested is in agreement with the published pharmacology; 5-HT > 1-(m-Chlorophenyl-) Piperazine hydrochloride > 1-(1-Napthyl) Piperazine hydrochloride > Ketanserin tartarate = Clozapine *(2,3,8)*.

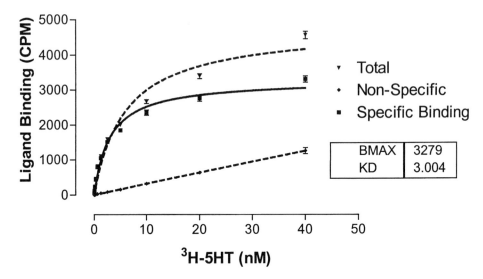

Fig. 4. Saturation binding of ^{3}H-5HT to $5HT_{2C}$ membranes: SPA format. Unlabeled 5-HT (10 μM), assay buffer and the indicated amounts of [^{3}H]-5HT ligand were added to 20 μg of $5HT_{2C}$ membranes, and the plates were incubated for 30 min at room temperature. 0.5 mg of WGA-PVT SPA beads were added, plates were mixed by shaking every 30 min for 2 h, and then counted in a MicroBeta (Wallac) counter as described in Materials and Methods. Each point represents the mean +/– SDM of quadruplicate determinations.

4.3. HTS Issues

11. In a typical HTS operation compounds are delivered already dissolved in DMSO, typically in the 1–10 mM range, and are then diluted into aqueous buffers to achieve the desired concentration for the screen. It is therefore important to define the DMSO tolerance of the assay (**Fig. 6**). The level of ^{3}H-5HT binding to 5-HT_{2C} membranes is unaffected by concentrations of DMSO less than 1.67%, but decreased significantly as the concentration of DMSO increased further (**Fig. 6**).

12. To generate sufficient amounts of membrane preparation for the HTS screen, a number of separate membrane lots were made from cell pastes harvested on different days. To ensure that these distinct membrane lots were of a consistent quality suitable for the HTS, displacement binding curves were run for each lot (**Fig. 7A**). Each of the 10 membrane lots tested exhibited overlapping homologous displacement binding curves (**Fig. 7A**), and therefore were judged acceptable.

13. In addition, since the HTS may be run over the period of several weeks and each membrane preparation may be used on several different days, stability to freeze-

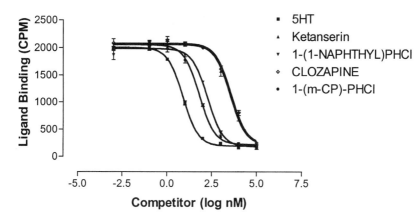

Fig. 5. Displacement binding of ^{3}H-5HT to $5HT_{2C}$ membranes. Unlabeled 5-HT, assay buffer, or competing compounds at the indicated concentrations, were incubated for 30 min at room temperature with 5 nM [^{3}H]-5HT and 20 μg of $5HT_{2C}$ membranes. 0.5 mg of WGA-PVT SPA beads were added, plates are mixed by shaking every 30 min for 2 h and then counted in a MicroBeta (Wallac) counter as described in Materials and Methods. Each point represents the mean +/– SDM of quadruplicate determinations.

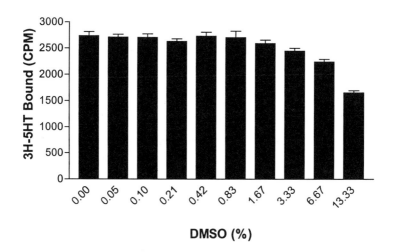

Fig. 6. DMSO tolerance. Unlabeled 5-HT (10 μM), or assay buffer with the indicated concentrations of DMSO were incubated for 30 min at room temperature with 5 nM [^{3}H]-5HT and 20 μg of $5HT_{2C}$ membranes. 0.5 mg of WGA-PVT SPA beads were added, plates were mixed by shaking every 30 min for 2 h and then counted in a MicroBeta (Wallac) counter as described in Materials and Methods. Each point represents the mean +/– SDM of quadruplicate determinations.

A

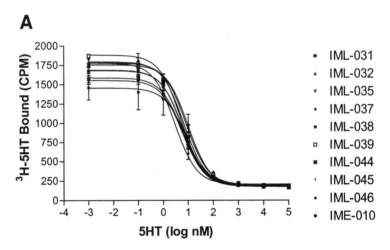

B

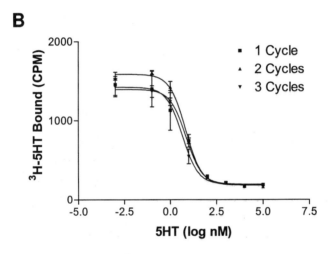

Fig. 7. Membrane quality control. (**A**) Comparison of membrane lots. Unlabeled 5-HT at the indicated concentrations or assay buffer were incubated for 30 min at room temperature with 5 n*M* [^{3}H]-5HT and 20 μg of the indicated lots of $5HT_{2C}$ membranes. 0.5 mg of WGA-PVT SPA beads were added, plates were mixed by shaking every 30 min for 2 h, and then counted in a MicroBeta (Wallac) counter as described in Materials and Methods. Each point represents the mean +/– SDM of quadruplicate determinations. (**B**) Stability to freeze-thaw. The assays were performed as described in 7A save that the $5HT_{2C}$ membranes used had been subjected to between 1 and 3 cycles of freeze-thaw, as indicated. Each point represents the mean +/– SDM of qua-druplicate determinations.

thaw is essential (**Fig. 7B**). The 5-HT$_{2C}$ membranes used in the HTS were found to be stable to at least three cycles of freeze-thaw, using a dry ice/ethanol bath to snap-freeze membranes (**Fig. 7B**).

14. It is also important to test reagent stability throughout a typical screening shift *(8)*. Typically all assay components are either maintained on ice or at ambient temperature, so the levels of total, specific, and nonspecific binding were determined over a 12-h period. For the 5-HT$_{2C}$ SPA assay, there did not appear to be any significant reagent stability issues under any of the conditions (data not shown), but because there appeared to be less variability in the data generated with reagents kept on ice, this procedure was adopted for the HTS process.

15. In the HTS process, competition for counter time from other assays or assays with sufficiently high throughput, may cause delays before counting. To assess the stability of the SPA-assay signal after incubation, plates may be counted at various times after the assay has been terminated. In general, SPA assays exhibit good signal stability for up to 24 h, and often beyond (data not shown).

4.4. Assay Window and Reproducibility

16. In order to rapidly identify the active compounds from the hundreds of thousands of compounds run in HTS, it is important that the assay be optimized to discriminate between active and inactive compounds *(4,21,22)*. The assay window, dynamic range, or the degree of separation between the background and maximum signals, should be both robust and reproducible *(21,22)*. Due to the nature of the procedure and the perturbation introduced by automation and human-associated random error all assay measurements contain a degree of variability, and it is in the context of this assay variability that active compounds must be distinguished from inactive compounds *(21,22)*. The lower the assay variability the higher the degree of confidence that an activity is "real" and will confirm upon re-testing *(21,22)*.

17. To address these assay window and reproducibility issues for the 5-HT$_{2C}$ binding SPA, two full 96-well plates for maximum binding and nonspecific binding were run on three separate days (**Fig. 8**). There is a robust separation of the total and nonspecific binding responses on all three days, and the variability associated with these signals produced signal windows of between 5 and 10 standard deviations on all three days, indicating that the 5-HT$_{2C}$ binding SPA is very good for HTS.

4.5. HTS Data

18. In the primary screen 150,000 compounds were tested in singlet wells at a final concentration of 10 μM and 0.5% DMSO (**Table 1**). A total of 2,752 compounds were identified as active because they inhibited ^{3}H-5HT binding by >/= 50%, producing an overall active rate of 1.83% (**Table 1**).

19. Colored compounds with absorption maxima in the 400–450 nm range (red, yellow, or orange) will absorb or quench the emitted light from the SPA bead and

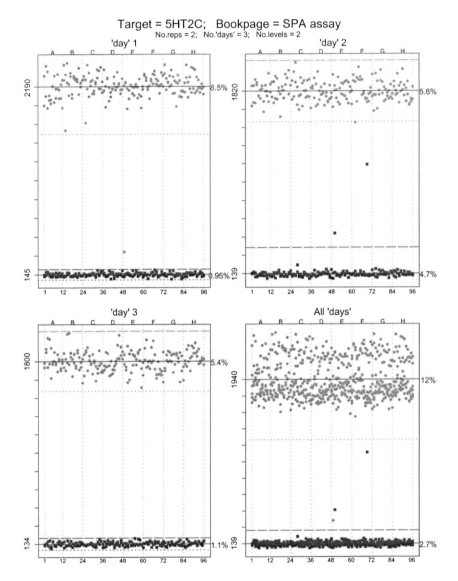

Fig. 8. Assay window and reproducibility. Unlabeled 5-HT (10 μ*M*), or assay buffer, were incubated for 30 min at room temperature with 5 n*M* [³H]-5HT and 20 μg of 5HT$_{2C}$ membranes. 0.5 mg of WGA-PVT SPA beads were added, plates were mixed by shaking every 30 min for 2 h and then counted in a MicroBeta (Wallac) counter as described in Materials and Methods. Two full 96-well plates for maximum binding and nonspecific binding (+10 μ*M* unlabeled 5-HT) were run on three separate days. The data are represented on a separate scattergram (2 plates of max and min signals) for each of the 3 d, together with a combined scattergram (6 plates of max and min signals) for all 3 d.

Table 1
5-HT$_{2C}$ Receptor Binding HTS Summary[a]

| | 5-HT$_{2C}$ Binding SPA HTS Summary | | | |
| | Primary Assay | | IC$_{50}$ Confirmation | |
Compound source	# Tested	Rapid actives*	IC$_{50}$ actives*	% Confirmed actives
Combinatorial chemistry	115,311	1465	1176	1.02
Organic file	35,391	1287	988	2.79
Total	150,702	2752	2164	1.44

[a]Active compounds inhibited 5-HT$_{2C}$ binding by >/=%, and were confirmed to inhibit 5-HT$_{2C}$ binding >/= 50% in a 5-point 10-fold dilution IC$_{50}$ assay.

can lead to false-positives in an inhibitor assay. The problem can be corrected by minimizing the concentration of the test compound, or by utilizing a color-quench correction curve specific for the counter used.

20. In 5-point 10-fold dilution IC$_{50}$ confirmation assays, 2,164 of these compounds were confirmed to inhibit ^{3}H-5HT binding by >/= 50%, producing an overall confirmation rate of 78.6% (**Table 1**), indicating that the SPA format was highly reproducible.

21. The primary screen of 150,000 compounds, and IC$_{50}$ assays to confirm active compounds were completed in a period of 12 wk, indicating that the SPA format supports HTS.

22. A number of structural platforms were identified with sufficient potency that they were further evaluated in a variety of secondary assays, indicating that the SPA format HTS was successful.

4.6. Conclusions

The SPA methodology for receptor-binding assays provides a number of benefits for HTS. The homogeneous format eliminates the need for a separation step, can be completely automated using robotic liquid handlers, reduces the number of operators required to run the assay, and thereby increases throughput. The homogeneous SPA format eliminates the need for addition of liquid scintillant and minimizes both the exposure of personnel to radioactive liquids and the amount of radioactive waste generated. The recent trends in HTS are to reduce costs and increase throughput by assay miniaturization, in which assays are carried out in smaller volumes using high-density well arrays of 384-, 864- and 1536-well plates. 384 well format assays have been developed using SPA technology and conventional PMT-based scintillation counters, but the time required to count plates becomes a rate-limiting step. Recent developments with new fluor-containing particles and charged coupled device (CCD) camera-based imaging systems should provide a means to con-figure radioligand receptor-binding assays compatible with 96-well and higher-density arrays to provide higher throughputs, and potentially reduce costs. In addition to the SPA bead format discussed here there are also microtiter plate proximity-based options (FlashPlate® [New England Nuclear] and Cytostar T™ [Amersham]) available for radioligand binding assays. The basic principles are similar to the fluomicrosphere technology, in that receptors of interest can be attached to the scintillant coated or impregnated plates by a variety of passive coating or coupling procedures, and the assay is a simple matter of adding radioligand with test compound, incubation, and measurement. Continued innovation in the fields of SPA technology, signal-capture instru-mentation, and automation will ensure that radioligand-binding assays will continue to be the mainstay of HTS, drug discovery, and drug development.

References

1. Cook, N. D. (1996) Scintillation proximity assay: a versatile high-throughput screening technology. *Drug Discovery Today* **1(7)**, 287–294.
2. Baez, M., Kursar, J. D., Helton, L. A., Wainscott, D. B., and Nelson, L. G. (1995) Molecular biology of serotonin receptors. *Obesity Res.* **3(Suppl. 4)**, 441S–447S.
3. Lucaites, V. L., Nelson, D. L., Wainscott, D. B., and Baez, M. (1996) Receptor subtype and density determine the coupling repertoire of the 5-HT2 receptor sub-family. *Life Sci.* **59(13)**, 1081–1095.
4. Lutz, M. W., Menius, J. A., Choi, T. D., Laskody, R. G., Domanico, P. L., Goetz, A. S, and Saussy, D. L. (1996) Experimental design for high-throughput screening. *Drug Discovery Today* **1(7)**, 277–286.
5. Major, J. S. (1995) Challenges of high throughput screening against cell surface receptors. *J. Receptor Signal Transd. Res.* **15(1–4)**, 595–607.
6. Janssen, M. J., Ensing, K., and de Zeeuw, R. A. (1999) Improved benzodiazepine radioreceptor assay using the multiscreen® assay system. *J. Pharmaceut. Biomed. Anal.* **20**, 753–761.
7. Froidevaux, S, Meier, M., Häusler, M., Macke, H., Beglinger, C., and Eberle, A. N. (1999) A microplate binding assay for the somatostatin type-2 receptor (SSTR2). *J. Receptor Signal Transd. Res.* **19(1–4)**, 167–180.
8. Kahl, S. D., Hubbard, F. R., Sittampalam, G. S., and Zock, J. M. (1997) Valida-tion of a high throughput scintillation proximity assay for 5-hydroxytryptamine$_{1E}$ receptor binding activity. *J. Biomol. Screening* **2(1)**, 33–40.
9. Bosworth, N. and Towers, P. (1989) Scintillation proximity assay. *Nature* **341**, 167–168.
10. Bylund, D. B. and Toews, M. L. (1993) Radioligand binding methods: practical guide and tips. *Am. J. Physiol.* **265**(*Lung Cell. Mold Physiol. 9*) L421–L429.
11. Rovati, G. E. (1993) Rational experimental design and data analysis for ligand binding studies tricks, tips and pitfalls. *Pharmacol. Res.* **28(4)**, 297–299.

12. Keen, M. (1995) The problems and pitfalls of radioligand binding. (1995) *Methods Mol. Biol.* **41,** 1–16.
13. Banks, P., Gosselin, M., and Prystay, L. (2000) Fluorescence Polarization Assays for high throughput screening of G protein-coupled receptors. *J. Biomol. Screening* **5(3),** 159–167.
14. Allen, M., Reeves, J., and Mellor, G. (2000) High throughput fluorescence polarization: a homogeneous alternative to radioligand binding for cell surface receptors. *J. Biomol. Screening* **5(2),** 63–69.
15. Qume, M. (1999) Overview of ligand-receptor binding tecniques. *Methods Mol. Biol.* **106,** 3–23.
16. Keen, M. (1999) Definition of receptors in radioligand-binding experiments. *Methods Mol. Biol.* **106,** 187–196.
17. Schumacher, C. and von Tscharner, V. (1994) Practical instructions for radioactively labeled ligand receptor binding studies. *Anal. Biochem.* **222,** 262–269.
18. Wahlström, A. (1978) Methodological aspects on drug receptor binding analysis. *Acta Pharmacol. Toxicol.* **43(11),** 74–78.
19. Roessler, N., Englert, D., and Neumann, K. (1993) New instruments for high throughput receptor binding assays. *J. Receptor Res.* **13(1–4),** 135–145.
20. Cusack, B. and Richelson, E. (1993) A method for radioligand binding assays using a robotic workstation. *J. Receptor Res.* **13(1–4),** 123–134.
21. Sittampalam, G. S, Iversen, P. W., Boadt, J. A., Kahl, S. D., Bright, S., Zock, J. M., et al. (1997) Design of signal windows in high throughput screening assays for drug discovery. *J. Biomol. Screening* **2(3),** 159–169.
22. Zhang, J. H., Chung, T. D. Y, and Oldenburg, K. R. (1999) A simple statistical parameter for use in evaluation and validation of high throughput screening assays. *J. Biomol. Screening* **4(2),** 67–73.

3

Homogeneous Techniques for Monitoring Receptor–Ligand Interactions

James S. Marks, Douglas S. Burdette, and David A. Giegel

1. Introduction

Radioligand binding is a well-established technique that has been used to study the interactions of extracellular ligands and their corresponding cell-surface receptors *(1)*. The initial studies relied on laborious, vacuum-filtration techniques that are cumbersome and difficult to automate. Despite these limitations, filtration-based radioligand binding assays were adequate to probe the kinetics of receptor-ligand interactions and to screen small libraries of compounds in search of receptor-binding antagonists. A number of reviews are available that described this methodology in detail *(2,3)*.

Recent technological advances have dramatically changed the logistics of drug discovery. Thanks to advances in both combinatorial chemistry and genomics, the number of compounds available for screening has increased by at least an order of magnitude and the number of targets presented to the high-throughput screening (HTS) lab is expected to increase on the order of two- to threefold. These changes have forced drug-screening scientists to seek out new technologies that dramatically increase throughput at reasonable costs.

Filtration assays are nonhomogeneous, because they rely on component separation. They typically require liquid handling steps both to initiate the assay and after reaction completion. Scintillation proximity assay (SPA) technology (Amersham-Pharmacia; Uppsala, Sweden) provided a homogeneous screening approach that eliminated the post-reaction liquid handling steps. The SPA system is well-uited to HTS and automation since it requires only the combining of assay reagents to generate the signal. In SPA, an isotope such as ^3H or ^{125}I is brought very close to a scintillant-impregnated bead by binding to its surface. Because the emitted beta particles or augur electrons travel short

From: *Methods in Molecular Biology, vol. 190: High Throughput Screening: Methods and Protocols*
Edited by: W. P. Janzen © Humana Press Inc., Totowa, NJ

distances in the bulk solution, the beads preferentially capture electrons from the bound radiolabeled ligand. Therefore, the amount of light emitted from the scintillant in the bead is directly proportional to the amount of bound, radiolabeled ligand. Beads coated with wheat germ agglutinin (WGA) bind cell membranes with high affinity through membrane surface carbohydrates. The amount of radiolabeled ligand bound to a membrane receptor can then be monitored by scintillation intensity from the bead. Compounds that interfere with or that enhance the receptor-ligand interaction are detected by alterations in the scintillation signal. This contrasts with the liquid transfers and multiple wash steps in a typical vacuum-filtration assay design. However, both the technical details of performing an assay and the applicability of the assay format are critical to successful automation and high assay throughput. The ongoing reassessment of technologies that will meet the throughput needs of modern drug discovery would therefore benefit from real-world comparisons of screening results from various assay types. These comparisons should include the newer homogeneous technologies like SPA and traditional assay methods like vacuum filtration.

This review presents a case study of one receptor-binding assay that initially utilized vacuum-filtration to separate bound from free ligand, and later was converted to a Scintillation Proximity Assay (Amersham Pharmacia Biotech) format, obviating the need for this separation step. Converting to SPA enabled us to automate the screen, thus increasing throughput two to fourfold. In addition, this methodology is amenable to miniaturization, which should enable us to conserve reagents and compound supplies, while minimizing waste.

Finally, there are a number of emerging technologies that are applicable to receptor-binding assays. While we will focus on one particular case study that employed SPA, we will also briefly discuss a few alternative techniques. The reason for this is that no one strategy will be successful in all circumstances and it is better to have as many tools as possible in an assay toolbox in order to increase the probability of success.

2. Materials

1. Ligand: Unlabeled ligand used in these studies was commercially available. The radioiodinated form was custom labeled for us by Dupont NEN (Boston, MA).

2.1. Preparation of Plasma Membranes

1. Lysis buffer (5 mM HEPES, pH 7.5, 2 mM etylenediamineteraacetic acid [EDTA], 5 μg/mL leupeptin, 5 μg/mL aprotinin, 5 μg/mL chymostatin, and 100 μg/mL phenylmethlysulfonylfluoride [PMSF]).

2. Storage buffer (10 mM HEPES, pH 7.5, 300 mM sucrose, 1 µg/mL leupeptin, 1 µg/mL aprotinin, 1 µg/mL chymostatin, and 100 µg/mL PMSF).

2.2. Ligand-Binding Assay: Vacuum Filtration

1. Binding buffer (10 mM HEPES, pH 7.2, 1 mM CaCl$_2$, 5 mM MgCl$_2$, and 0.5% bovine serum albumin [BSA]).
2. GF/c glass-fiber filtermat (PerkinElmer Wallac Inc., Gaithersburg, MD).
3. Wash buffer (binding buffer supplemented with 0.5 M NaCl).
4. Microbeta Scintillation Counter (PerkinElmer Wallac).

2.3. Ligand-Binding Assay: Scintillation Proximity Assay

1. White, clear-bottom 96-well microtiter plates.
2. Assay buffer: 10 mM HEPES, pH 7.2, 1 mM CaCl$_2$, 5 mM MgCl$_2$, and 0.5 % (w/v) BSA.
3. WGA-coated SPA beads (Cat. no. RPNQ0011; Amersham-Pharmacia).
4. Dimethylsulfoxide (DMSO).
5. Trilux 1450 Microbeta scintillation counter (PerkinElmer Wallac).
6. Serum-supplemented Hank's medium.
7. Coulter Counter (Beckman Coulter, Inc., Fullerton, CA, USA).
8. Multidrop (TiterTek Instruments, Huntsville, AL, USA).

3. Methods
3.1. Preparation of Plasma Membranes

1. Receptors used in these studies were prepared from THP-1 cells.
2. Approximately 1×10^8 cells were washed in Dulbecco's phosphate-buffered saline (PBS) and homogenized with a dounce homogenizer in 25 mL of lysis buffer.
3. The homogenate was then centrifuged at 750g and 4°C for 10 min and the supernatant was centrifuged a second time for 30 min at 4°C at 25,000g.
4. The resultant pellet was resuspended in storage buffer to a protein concentration of 1–2 mg/mL and immediately frozen at –80°C.

3.2. Ligand-Binding Assay: Vacuum Filtration

1. The reaction was performed by incubating ^{125}I-ligand (0.2 pM) and 20 µg membrane protein in binding buffer at room temperature for 30 min.
2. Nonspecific ligand binding was assessed by performing the assay in the presence of a 100-fold excess of cold ligand.
3. The reaction was terminated by filtering the contents of each well onto a GF/c glass-fiber filtermat and each well was washed with a total of 600 µL of ice-cold wash buffer.
4. The filters were allowed to dry for approx 30 min in a 37°C oven, and then sealed in a clear plastic bag that contained enough scintillation cocktail to saturate the filter. The filters were then counted using a Microbeta Scintillation Counter.

3.3. Ligand-Binding Assay: Scintillation Proximity Assay

3.3.1. Receptor-Ligand Membrane Assay

1. This receptor-ligand membrane assay was run in white, clear-bottom 96-well microtiter plates with a final volume per well of 200 µL.
2. Each reaction contained assay buffer, 6 µg/mL receptor containing membranes, 2.5 mg/mL WGA-coated SPA beads, 35 pM ^{125}I labeled ligand, and 1% (v/v) DMSO.
3. Nonspecific binding was determined by adding a 100-fold excess of cold ligand to specific control wells.
4. Inhibitors were added to the plate in 2 µL of DMSO prior to other assay components.
5. Plates were sealed, assay components were mixed by inversion, and the plates were incubated at room temperature (25°C) for 4 h prior to scintillation detection using a Trilux 1450 Microbeta scintillation counter.

3.3.2. Whole-Cell Assays

1. Whole-cell assays, like the membrane assays, were performed in white, clear-bottom 96-well microtiter plates with a final volume per well of 200 µL.
2. Cells were grown in serum-supplemented Hank's medium and culture cell densities were determined with a Coulter Counter (Beckman Coulter).
3. The cells and ligand were diluted to the appropriate concentrations in assay buffer and added to the reaction using a multidrop (TiterTek Instruments). Whole cell reactions were also run in the presence of 1% DMSO.

3.4. Results and Discussion

In order to meet the challenge of screening many more samples against an increasing number of therapeutic targets, there must be an almost symbiotic relationship between automation and biology. Techniques requiring manual intervention or that are difficult to automate are being replaced by newer, automation-amenable, homogeneous methodologies. Receptor-binding assays have been among the most difficult types of screens to automate, due to the amount of manual intervention that is attached to the standard method, vacuum filtration. Automating the assay prior to the vacuum-filtration step is straightforward. However, the postreaction sample processing steps are very laborious and time consuming. The contents of each plate are filtered onto a coded filtermat and then the mats are dried, soaked in scintillation cocktail, and sealed in a plastic bag prior to scintillation counting. Large quantities of wash buffer are also required. Despite its drawbacks, this technique is perfectly adequate for processing six to seven thousand samples a day and it enabled us to screen a 10^5 sample collection in a reasonable period of time.

The number of samples in the average compound library has increased dramatically in the last 10 yr. While adequate to screen 10^5 compounds, vacuum filtration is far too cumbersome when screening collections approaching 10^6 samples. SPA technology provided scientists with an assay format that obviated the need to separate bound from free ligand and was amenable to automation. Briefly, isolated receptors, usually in the form of plasma-membrane fragments, are incubated in the presence of labeled ligand, scintillant-impregnated, polyvinlytoluene, or yttrium-silicate beads that are coated with WGA, and test compound. The applicability of the technique rests with the attraction between the lectin on the surface of the beads and specific carbohydrate moieties on the surface of the plasma-membrane vesicles. If the beads and membranes are compatible, then the receptor-laden membranes coat the beads and the ligand then can be detected once it combines with its receptor. Thus, receptor-binding inhibitors, for example, can be detected by their ability to prevent the labeled ligand from binding to its receptor.

3.5. Other Homogeneous Technologies

In the past few years, a number of new homogeneous technologies have been introduced that enable scientists to miniaturize their receptor binding assays and take better advantage of their automated workstations. Leadseeker (AP Biotech), a second-generation SPA methodology, is an example of one such technology. It operates along the same lines as the original SPA, but incorporates two significant improvements that increases sensitivity while reducing detection time. First, a new species of bead has been introduced that fluoresces in the red region (660 nm) of the spectrum in the presence of a beta particle or auger electron. Second, these beads are used in conjunction with a new CCD-based detector that operates most efficiently in the same region of the spectrum in which the beads fluoresce. The reduction in detection time is due to the fact that the camera images the entire plate at one time, rather than one or even multiple wells at a time.

Table 1 compares the throughput of a hypothetical assay as you increase plate density and decrease assay volume. If one assumes that an individual is capable of processing approx 100 plates a day in a conventional filtration assay, then converting to an SPA format immediately increases throughput almost threefold. Interestingly, converting the assay to a format that is compatible with 384-well microplates, does not significantly affect throughput due to throughput limitations of current detectors. It is not until you change detection methods (e.g., Leadseeker) and use 384-well plates, that you enjoy the full benefit of SPA technology. In addition to attaining throughput numbers that meet the criteria for ultra-high throughput screening, lowering the assay volume to 25 μL for 384-well plates also reduces waste and helps to conserve the compound collection.

Table 1
Effect of SPA and Leadseeker on Screening Throughput

	Conventional SPA		Leadseeker SPA	
Output parameters	96	384	96	384
Read time per plate (min)	5	20	5	5
Plates day/person	288	72	288	288
Data points day/person	27,648	27,648	27,648	110,592

In addition to SPA, a number of other homogeneous technologies have been introduced that are amenable to receptor-binding assays. These include reporter genes *(4)*, fluorescence polarization, and fluorescence correlation spectroscopy, just to name a few. Fluorescence polarization is one such method that has been applied to a number of cell-surface receptors, including vasopressin (V1a), β_1-adrenergic receptor, and 5-HT$_3$ *(5)*. This methodology is uniquely suited to measure these types of interactions because it measures the ratio of bound to free ligand. It is based on two principles *(9)*: (1) fluorescent molecules will emit light in the same polarized plane, if the molecule does not rotate during the interval between excitation and emission; and (2) due to energy and momentum considerations, smaller molecules rotate faster than larger molecules at the same temperature. In this type of assay plane polarized light is used for fluorescence excitation. The unbound fluoropeptide rotates rapidly in solution and emits light equally in all directions. Upon binding to the much larger receptor, the ligand's rotation rate slows. This increases the amount of light emitted in the same plane as that used for excitation and thus, the assay signal also increases.

The utility of this technique had been limited by the availability of suitable microplate readers. In the last five years, however, a number of companies have introduced multifunctional detectors that remedy this situation. **Table 2** lists some of the multifunctional detectors that are available with which we have some experience. This list was not meant to be all-inclusive, nor was there any attempt to rank these detectors in order of preference.

Finally, fluorescence correlation spectroscopy (FCS) can be used to monitor homogeneous receptor binding assays at potentially very small volumes. This technique uses confocal optics to illuminate a small portion of the total well. FCS, like fluorescence polarization, is predicated on the fact that small fluorophores behave differently than large fluorophores. In FCS, however, it is not the degree to which emitted light is polarized that is measured, rather it is the relative rate of translational mobility that is monitored. Simply stated, smaller molecules move faster than large molecules at the same temperature,

Table 2
Comparison of High Density Multifunctional Plate Readers

Product name	Manufacturer	Supported plate formats	Detection technology	F	TRF	FP	Lum	Abs	Radio
Analyst	LjL Biosystems	96/384	PMT	●	●	●	●	●	
Acquest	LjL Biosystems	384/1536	PMT	●	●	●	●	●	
Fusion	Packard Instr.	96/384/1536	PMT	●	●		●	●	
Leadseeker	Amersham	<= 1536	CCD	●					●
Polarstar	BMG	96/384/1536	PMT	●	●	●	●	●	
Ultra	Tecan	96/384/1536	PMT	●	●	●	●	●	
Victor^2 V	PerkinElmer	96/384/1536	PMT	●	●	●	●	●	
ViewLux	PerkinElmer	<= 2000	CCD	●	●		●	●	

and so they spend less time in the confocal volume. This means that the total fluorescence emitted by small species as they travel through a defined volume is, on average, much less than that emitted by a larger, slower species that spends appreciably more time in the confocal volume. There are a number of reviews available *(7,8)* that provide a good overview of FCS and other fluorescent techniques.

In summary, a number of homogeneous methodologies are now available that are suitable for performing receptor-binding assays. While the original vacuum-filtration technique was adequate for characterizing small sample databases, these new technologies are better suited for screening many more compounds, and in smaller assay volumes.

4. Notes

1. It would be useful to pause here, and consider the steps necessary to convert an assay from vacuum filtration to SPA. SPA development workflow is similar to that for any other assay type but it requires consideration of components unique to SPA signal detection.
2. The first step involves setting up a multiparametric experiment that is based around the best estimates of conditions (**Table 3**). Because of their widespread historical use, conditions employed in typical filtration experiments are often used to estimate initial assay conditions.
3. The amount of WGA-coated beads per well, the concentration of labeled ligand, and the amount of membrane protein are all varied in the presence and absence of saturating concentrations of cold ligand. **Table 4** lists the results generated by this experiment and indicates the optimal assay conditions. In this case, 1 mg beads, 35 pM radioligand, and 1.24 μg membrane preparation per well yielded a consistent signal to noise ratio in excess of 10-fold with reasonable amounts of material.
4. Having established the conditions for a viable assay, other HTS adaptation parameters can be examined. Factors including tolerance to DMSO, stability of the reactants under conditions the screening conditions, and the extent to which the assay can be miniaturized must be addressed prior to running an HTS screen.
5. It is necessary to determine the viability of the test reagents in order to determine the number of plates that comprise a single run, and the most appropriate means of automating an assay.
6. In our lab, we utilize isolated stand-alone workstations with stackers as well as fully automated, turnkey systems.
7. Our example assay tolerates up to 4% (v/v) DMSO, with > 12-h stability of reagent stocks stored on ice and the signal remains stable for > 24-h.
8. Finally, it is important to establish that the results attained are independent of the method used. Accordingly, two known inhibitors were titrated (**Fig. 1**) against ^{125}I-labeled ligand in an effort to verify that the IC_{50} values obtained with this technique were similar to values obtained with the filtration technique.
9. The standard IC_{50} equation provided an excellent fit to the SPA data.

Table 3
Raw Data from SPA Matrix Trial

	Beads (mg/well)	^{125}I-Ligand (pM)	Cold ligand	Protein (μg/well)						
				0	1.24	2.48	4.96	9.92	14.88	24.8
1	0.5	35	−	100	1431	2229	990	1271	850	673
2	0.5	70	−	208	3083	2045	2013	2502	2041	1319
3	0.5	140	−	289	3637	1768	2999	3653	2999	2193
4	1	35	−	164	2410	2133	1684	1387	1447	1163
5	1	70	−	317	4131	3067	5672	4558	3176	2646
6	1	140	−	581	3918	4058	5057	6546	5607	4407
7	2	35	−	233	1776	2791	2466	2823	2085	2133
8	2	70	−	573	3649	678	1568	5478	5879	5374
9	2	140	−	1075	6177	8348	10,834	8789	10,024	8977
10	0.5	35	+	92	305	232	293	289	253	285
11	0.5	70	+	321	589	701	613	633	605	645
12	0.5	140	+	281	790	1094	1279	934	1275	1030
13	1	35	+	172	297	353	493	553	581	597
14	1	70	+	273	878	882	1135	1179	1090	1155
15	1	140	+	613	882	1383	1860	1592	1527	1872
16	2	35	+	289	525	609	625	714	742	950
17	2	70	+	569	994	1315	1487	1748	1780	2117
18	2	140	+	1018	1866	1977	2293	2679	2671	1259

Table 4
Signal to Noise Ratio

Beads (mg/well)	^{125}I-Ligand (pM)	Cold ligand	Protein (µg/well)					
			1.24	2.48	4.96	9.92	14.88	24.8
0.5	35	–	6.2	**15.2**	4.4	5.9	4.7	3.0
0.5	70	–	**10.7**	4.8	6.2	7.4	6.5	3.4
0.5	140	–	6.6	1.8	2.7	5.2	2.7	2.5
1	35	–	**18.0**	10.9	4.7	3.2	3.1	2.4
1	70	–	6.3	4.5	6.2	4.7	3.5	2.6
1	140	–	**12.4**	4.5	3.6	6.1	5.5	3.0
2	35	–	6.5	8.0	6.6	6.1	4.1	2.9
2	70	–	7.2	0.1	1.1	4.2	4.4	3.1
2	140	–	6.0	7.6	7.7	4.6	5.4	32.8

10. The IC$_{50}$ values calculated from the SPA titrations were within twofold of those determined by filtration. Therefore, the SPA assay measured the targeted biochemical activity, provided comparable results to those for the reference assay, and demonstrated a similar ability to identify receptor-ligand interaction antagonists.

11. Once adapted to this homogeneous technology, this receptor-binding assay could leverage the efficiencies of automation. Fully automating the screen reduced by >50% the required personnel time, freeing a highly trained colleague for other work during the screen. Miniaturizing the assay through reduced total assay volume and running in 384-well plates added to the time and resource savings.

12. There has been a debate within the research community concerning the pros and cons of screening using isolated membranes vs whole cells. From a logistical standpoint, it is preferable to screen with isolated membranes because you can prepare and store large quantities of a single batch in advance of the screen. This reduces the overall variation in the data, ensures that adequate quantities of the receptor are on hand prior the initiation of the screen, and increases your signal by effectively enriching your receptor population.

13. While convenient for screening, it must be pointed out that during the isolation procedure, the receptor is subjected to high shear forces, nonphysiological conditions, and could potentially be separated from cytoplasmic effectors that influence ligand binding and physiological function. Indeed, it has been our experience that while the confirmed hit profiles obtained using whole cells vs isolated membranes overlap almost completely, each can contain unique compounds. Thus, a case can be made in favor of both screen types.

14. For the reasons outlined earlier, it was decided to attempt a whole-cell scintillation proximity assay. Except for a few brief technical reports from AP Biotech, no reports of whole cell SPA screens were identified. This raised a question of SPA format suitability for whole cell screens.

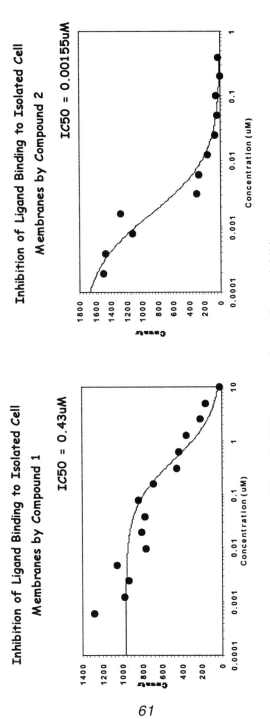

Fig. 1. Inhibition curves for two known inhibitors.

Table 5
Receptor-Binding Assay Utilizing SPA Technology and Whole Cells

Culture media	Condition	0.125 mg WGA SPA beads/well		0.5 mg WGA beads/well	
		100,000 cells/well	500,000 cells/well	100,000 cells/well	500,000 cell/well
HEPES	Total	2065 ± 454	2989 ± 476	2703 ± 346	4957 ± 682
	Nonspecific	281 ± 33	720 ± 63	777 ± 250	1101 ± 336
HEPES + NaCl (120 mM)	Total	542 ± 25	1025 ± 242	858 ± 266	1729 ± 61
	Nonspecific	152 ± 25	291 ± 18	253 ± 4	325 ± 198
RPMI	Total	346 ± 154	508 ± 62	560 ± 234	1091 ± 137
	Nonspecific	87 ± 25	160 ± 33	185 ± 45	309 ± 69
PBS	Total	1174 ± 257	800 ± 196	842 ± 50	1384 ± 59
	Nonspecific	147 ± 10	355 ± 22	284 ± 60	673 ± 16

15. While not straightforward, conditions for a whole-cell SPA were identified (**Table 5**). Factors including salt concentration and species had a profound impact on assay signal and signal stability over time adding complexity to the optimization process. At 10^5 cells/well and a bead concentration of 0.125 mg/well, we observed a signal to noise ratio of approx 7. The magnitude of the window was very much in line with the results from the membrane SPA.

16. FACS experiments confirmed that the cells remained viable under the assay conditions (data not shown).

17. While this format introduced problems of obtaining and maintaining sufficient viable cells to feed the screen, whole cell SPAs appear to be viable.

References

1. Fernandes, P. B. (1998) Technological advances in high-throughput screening. *Curr. Opin. Chem. Biol.* **2,** 597–603.

2. Bylund, D. B. and Yamamura, H. I. (1990) Methods for receptor binding, in Methods in Neurotransmitter Receptor Analysis (Yamamura, H. I., Enna, S. J., and Kuha, M. J., eds.), Raven Press, New York, NY pp. 1–35.

3. Qume, M. (1999) Overview of ligand-receptor binding techniques, in *Methods in Molecular Biology* (Keen, M., ed.), Humana Press Inc., Totowa, NJ, 3–23.

4. Zlokarnik, G., Negulescu, P.A., Knapp, T. E., Mere, L., Burres, N., Feng, L., et al. (1998) Quantitation of transcription and clonal selection of single living cells with B-lactamase as reporter. *Science* **279,** 84–88.

5. Allen, M., Reeves, J., and Mellor, G. (2000) High throughput fluorescence polarization: a homogeneous alternative to radioligand binding for cell surface receptors. *J. Biomol. Screening* **5,** 63–69.

6. Parker, G. J., Law, T. L., Lenoch, F. J., and Bolger, R. E. (2000) Development of high throughput screening assays using fluorescence polarization: nuclear receptor-ligand-binding and kinase/phosphatase assays. *J. Biomol. Screening* **5,** 77–88.

7. Moore, K. J., Turconi, S., Ashman, S., Ruediger, M., Haupts, U., Emerick, V., and Pope, A. J. (2000) Single molecule detection technologies in miniaturized high throughput screening: fluorescence correlation spectroscopy. *J. Biomol. Screening* **5,** 335–353.

8. Haupts, U., Rudiger, M., and Pope, A. J. (2000) Macroscopic versus microscopic fluorescence techniques in (ultra)-high throughput screening. *DDT:HTS* **(Suppl. 1),** 3–9

9. Atkins, P. W. (1994) Physical chemistry, 5th ed. W. H. Freeman Co., New York, NY, pp. 1–17.

4

Comparison of SPA, FRET, and FP for Kinase Assays

Jinzi J. Wu

1. Introduction

During the last few years, a variety of technologies have been developed for rapid discovery of protein kinase inhibitors from both synthetic small-molecule libraries and natural products *(1–8)*. Many of high throughput kinase assays have been developed in 96-, 384-, and 1536-well formats using these technologies *(9–11)*. Development of these technologies allow one to quickly large synthetic compound or natural product libraries in a very short period of time with high sensitivity, accuracy, and reproducibility. Therefore, development of these new technologies has significantly accelerated the process of discovering drug leads for kinases. In this chapter, I will summarize and compare a number of technologies for development of homogeneous, high-throughput kinase assays.

1.1. Scintillation Proximity Assays for Serine/Threonine Kinases

The scintillation proximity assay (SPA) technology has been used in the development of homogeneous assays for many molecular targets including kinases *(1,12–14)*. In this section, development and optimization of an SPA for a serine/threonine kinase, Cdk4, has been described. Cdk4 kinase activity has been shown to be misregulated in a majority of malignant cells *(15)*. Therefore, there is significant interest to identify selective Cdk4 inhibitors for cancer therapy. Discovery of Cdk4 inhibitors requires high-throughput and robust assays that would enable screening of hundreds of thousands of compounds in a short period of time. However, the assays reported in the literature for measurement of Cdk4 kinase activity *(16,17)* are not amenable to high-throughput screening (HTS). These published assays for Cdk4 often use $[\gamma\text{-}^{32}P]ATP$ or $[\gamma\text{-}^{33}P]ATP$ as a tracer, and a protein or synthetic peptide as a substrate. After

From: *Methods in Molecular Biology, vol. 190: High Throughput Screening: Methods and Protocols*
Edited by: W. P. Janzen © Humana Press Inc., Totowa, NJ

the phosphorylation reaction is carried out, the radiolabeled protein or peptide is then analyzed either by SDS-PAGE, thin layer chromatography (TLC), or by binding to a filter. Obviously, the SDS-PAGE or TLC method is very labor-intensive and not amenable to HTS. In the filter-binding, or filtration assay, separation of radiolabeled phosphoprotein or phosphopeptide from excess radioactive ATP is required after the phosphorylation reaction. This separation requires many steps, such as transferring the stopped reaction mixtures into a 96-well filtration plate followed by several washes with phosphoric acid. Furthermore, the plate has to be dried before scintillation liquid is added prior to counting in a liquid-scintillation counter. It is evident that this method is very time-consuming, not robotics-friendly, and difficult to apply to a HTS program.

I describe here the development of a novel homogeneous assay using an affinity peptide-tagging technology for rapidly discovering Cdk4 inhibitors. The DNA sequence encoding a streptavidin-recognition motif, or StrepTag (AWRHPQFGG) *(18)*, was cloned and expressed at the C-terminus of a fusion protein of a 152-amino acid hyperphosphorylation domain (Rb152) of the retinoblastoma protein (Rb) linked to GST at the N-terminus. This affinity peptide-tagged protein (GST-Rb152-StrepTag), which contains the two known phosphorylation sites of Rb, specifically phosphorylated by Cdk4 in vivo, was used as a substrate in the current in vitro kinase assay.

1.2. Fluorescence Resonance Energy Transfer Assays for Tyrosine Kinases

In the last few years, homogenous, time-resolved fluorescence resonance energy transfer (HTR-FRET) technology has been applied to the development of HTS assays for many molecular targets including tyrosine kinases *(4,19)*. This technology is based on FRET between two fluorescent labels, an energy donating long-lived label and a short-lived organic acceptor. The energy transfer occurs when the two labels are brought in close proximity via various molecular interactions. Since there are a few high-affinity anti-phosphotyrosine antibodies available commercially from PerkinElmer Wallac, (Gaithersburg, MD), Packard Instrument (Meriden, CT), and LJL BioSystems (Sunnyvale, CA), one can develop an HTR-FRET assay for tyrosine kinases using these antibodies. In general, europium chelate or cryptate labeled antiphosphotyrosine antibody serves as an energy donor and streptavidin-labeled allophycocyanin (APC) serves as an energy acceptor. Once biotinylated peptide or protein is phosphorylated by a tyrosine kinase, the donor and acceptor molecules are brought in close proximity via interactions of phosphotyrosine/antibody and biotin/streptavidin, and energy transfer occurs, generating a fluorescent signal at 665 nm. The HTR-FRET assay is sensitive, homogeneous, and quite tolerant to some extremes in reaction conditions. It is extremely useful for assay miniaturization. In this section, I compared different substrates and labeling technologies (chelate and cryptate) in development of tyrosine kinase assays.

1.3. Fluorescence Polarization Assays for Serine/Threonine Kinases

Fluorescence polarization (FP) has been applied to the development of robust, homogeneous, high-throughput assays in molecular-recognition research, such as ligand-protein interactions *(20,21)*. In principle, when fluorescently labeled small molecules in solution are excited by a polarized light source, the emission polarization can be affected by a number of mechanisms, the most predominate of which is rotational diffusion. For example, when a small fluorescently labeled ligand is bound to a high molecular-weight receptor, the complex will have a relatively slow rotational-diffusion rate, resulting in a high-emission polarization. When the ligand is displaced from the receptor molecule, it is free to rotate more quickly and consequently the emission is depolarized leading to a low-polarization signal. Therefore, competitors/inhibitors, which compete with the fluorescent ligand for the receptor, can be detected in solution in terms of a decrease in polarization. Recently, this technology has been applied to the development of homogeneous tyrosine kinase assays, since there are high-affinity antiphosphotyrosine antibodies available. Unlike tyrosine kinases, application of FP to assay development for serine/threonine kinases has been impeded due to lack of high-affinity antiphosphoserine/threonine antibodies. The conventional approaches for detection of serine/threonine kinase activities are nonhomogeneous such as radioactive PO_4-transfer assays. Recently, a homogeneous radioactive approach for serine/threonine kinases has been developed using SPA technology as described in the previous section. However, this approach generates radioactive waste and is not environmentally friendly.

I described here the discovery of a high-affinity antiphosphoserine antibody for the development of a simple, sensitive FP assay for serine/threonine kinases such as protein kinase C (PKC) in 384-well plates. Compared to the reported assays for serine/threonine kinases *(12,22,23)*, the FP assay is nonradioactive, homogeneous, robust and highly amenable to HTS.

2. Materials

2.1. Expression and Purification of GST-Rb152-StrepTag

1. Luria Bertani Media (LB).
2. Ampicillin.
3. pGEX4T-1 plasmid (Amersham Pharmacia).

4. Isopropyl-b-D-thiogalactopyranoside (IPTG)
5. Lysis buffer: 1X TBS, 1% NP40, 1 mM EDTA, 1 mM dithiotricitol (DTT), protease inhibitors (1 tablet Complete™, Behringer) in 50 mL, pH 8.0.
6. 40 mL column (2.6 × 8 cm) of glutathione-Sepharose 4B (Amersham Pharmacia).
7. Wash buffer: 20 mM Tris-HCl, 20 mM NaCl, 1 mM EDTA, 1 mM DTT, pH 8.0.
8. 10 mM reduced glutathione.
9. 1X PBS, 0.25 mM DTT.
10. Glycerol.

2.2. Scintillation Proximity Assay (SPA) for Serine/Threonine Kinases

2.2.1. Reagents and Supplies (SPA)

1. GST-Rb152.
2. GST-Rb152-StrepTag
3. [γ-^{33}P]ATP (specific activity = 2500 Ci/mmol, Amersham Pharmacia Biotech).
4. ATP.
5. 96-well microtiter plates (EG&G Wallac, Gaithersburg, MD).
6. Cdk4 buffer: Contains 25 mM MOPS, pH 7.2, 15 mM MgCl$_2$·6H$_2$O, 5 mM EGTA, 60 mM β-glycerophosphate, 0.1 mM sodium orthovanadate, 30 mM p-nitrophenyl phosphate, 1 mM DTT, and 0.2 µM okadaic acid (for stability purposes, the last three reagents were added on the day of the assay).
7. Stop buffer, containing 50 mM H$_3$PO$_4$, streptavidin- or glutathione-coated PVT SPA beads (cat. no. RPNQ.0007, Amersham Pharmacia Biotech), 50 mM ATP, 0.1% Triton-X.
8. Triton-X 100.

2.2.2. Equipment (SPA)

1. Sorvall HERMLE centrifuge (model RC-3B, Sorvall, Newton, CT).
2. 1450 MicroBeta liquid-scintillation counter (EG&G Wallac, Gaithersburg, MD).

2.3. Fluorescence Resonance Energy Transfer Assays for Tyrosine Kinases

2.3.1. Reagents and Supplies

1. 384-well OptiPlates (Packard Instruments Cooperation, CT).
2. Biotin-poly (Glu:Ala:Tyr) [6:3:1] and biotin-poly (Glu:Tyr) [4:1] (CIS Bio International, France).
3. Streptavidin xL-allophycocyanin conjugate (SA-xLAPC) were purchased from either CIS bio International or Prozyme Inc.
4. Europium cryptate labeled anti-phosphotyrosine antibody, PT66 (Packard Instruments).
5. Europium chelate-labeled PT66 was purchased from Wallac, Inc.
6. Assay buffer: 20 mM Tris-HCl, pH 7.5, 3 mM MgCl$_2$, and MnCl$_2$.
7. Buffer: 20 mM Tris-HCl, pH 7.5, 0.35% BSA, 35 mM EDTA, 1 M KF.

2.3.2. Equipment

1. Packard Discovery.
2. Wallac Victor 2.

2.4. Fluorescence Polarization Assays for Serine/Threonine Kinases

2.4.1. Reagents and Supplies

1. Black 96- or 384-well OptiPlates (cat. no. 6005256; Packard Instruments Cooperation).
2. HEPES, BGG (Bovine Gamma Globulin, Acetylated, cat. no. P2255), DTT (Dithiothreitol, catalog number P2032), and EDTA (cat. no. P2023) were purchased from Pan Vera Cooperation (Madison, WI) and these reagents are ultralow fluorescence-graded.
3. Seven commercially available antibodies were evaluated.
   a. Mouse monoclonal antiphosphoserine antibody V3156 (0.65 mg/mL) was purchased from Biomeda Corporation (Foster City, CA).
   b. Mouse polyclonal antiphosphoserine antibody V4156 was a gift from Biomeda Corporation.
   c. Mouse monoclonal antiphosphoserine antibody PSR-45 (5.3 mg/mL) (Research Diagnostics, Inc., Flanders, NJ).
   d. Monoclonal antiphosphoserine antibody PSG-45 (5.3 mg/mL) (Sigma, St. Louis, MO).
   e. Rabbit polyclonal antiphosphoserine antibody (3.3 mg/mL) was purchased from HTI Products (Ramona, CA).
   f. Rabbit polyclonal antiphosphoserine antibody against phosphoserine-21 in GSK3 was a gift from New England BioLabs or NEB (Beverly, MA).
   g. Mouse monoclonal antiphosphoserine antibody 2B9 (1 mg/mL) (Medical and Biological laboratory, Inc., Nagoya, Japan).
4. Three fluorescent peptide tracers (amides) were evaluated. They were designed in-house and custom-synthesized by SynPep Corporation (Dublis, CA).
   a. Fluorescein-Ahx-TSS(PO$_4$)FAEG (Ahx: 6-amino-hexanoic acid) or Tracer A.
   b. Fluorescein-GS(PO$_4$)FAEG or Tracer B.
   c. Fluorescein-RFARKGS(PO$_4$) LRQKNV or Tracer C.
   d. The fluorescein dye was purchased from Sigma.
5. The peptide substrates of PKC, fluorescein-RFARKGSLRQKNV (amide) and RFARKGSLRQKNV (amide), were custom-synthesized by SynPep Corporation.
6. PKCα (Pan Vera Corporation).
7. [γ-^{33}P]ATP (specific activity >2500 Ci/mmole) and streptavidin-coated PVT SPA beads (cat. no. RPNQ-0007) were purchased from Amersham Pharmacia Biotech.
8. FP buffer 1: 27 m*M* HEPES, pH 7.4, and 0.2 mg/mL BGG.
9. PKC buffer: 25 m*M* Tris-HCl, pH 7.4, 3 m*M* MgCl$_2$, and 2 m*M* CaCl$_2$.

2.4.2. Equipment

1. Analyst (LJL BioSystems Inc., Sunnyvale, CA).
2. 1450 MicroBeta liquid scintillation counter (EGRG Wallac, Gaithersburg, MD).

3. Methods

3.1. Expression and Purification of GST-Rb152-StrepTag

1. A volume of 50 mL LB, containing 100 μg/mL, was inoculated with a single colony of BL21(DE3), a strain of *Escherichia coli*, that bears a plasmid encoding the *GST-Rb152-StrepTag* fusion gene. The plasmid used was derived from pGEX4T-1 derivative.
2. The cells were grown overnight at 37°C.
3. Subsequently, 10 mL of the preculture was inoculated in 790 mL LB containing 100 μg/mL ampicillin.
4. The flasks were incubated at 30°C until the optical density (OD) of the culture (A_{600}) reached a value of 0.8–1.
5. Protein expression was induced at 23°C by adding 0.4 mM IPTG.
6. After centrifugation, the bacterial pellet was resuspended in 25 mL ice-cold lysis buffer.
7. The cells were lysed by passing three times through a French press (1000 psi). A clear supernatant was obtained after passing through 0.45-μm filters.
8. The lysates from 12 of these cultures were applied at 2 mL/min to a 40 mL column (2.6 × 8 cm) of glutathione-Sepharose 4B pre-equilibrated in lysis buffer.
9. The column was washed to base-line with lysis buffer (without the protease inhibitors) followed by 8 column volumes of wash buffer.
10. Absorbed GST-Rb152-StrepTag was finally eluted with wash buffer that contained 10 mM reduced glutathione.
11. The peak fraction was pooled and dialyzed overnight against 1 L of 1X PBS, 0.25 mM DTT. After dialysis, glycerol was added to a final concentration of 30%, the solution was aliquoted and stored at –80°C. Typical yields were 500–600 mg of a mixture of purified proteins that contain at least 70% of GST-Rb152-StrepTag fusion protein.

3.2. Scintillation Proximity Assay (SPA)

SPA technology was used for detection of the Cdk4 kinase activity. GST-Rb152, a biotinylated peptide (TRPPTLS × PIPHIPR) or GST-Rb152-StrepTag was used as a substrate in the assay (*see* **Notes 1** and **2**). [γ-^{33}P]ATP (specific activity = 2500 Ci/mmol) was used as a tracer. The assay was performed in 96-well microtiter plates in a final volume of 50 μL of Cdk4 buffer.

1. To start a reaction, Cdk4 was added into wells of a 96-well plate that already contained substrate, [γ-^{33}P]ATP, and ATP. The concentrations of Cdk4, substrate, [γ-^{33}P]ATP and ATP are indicated in the text or figure legends.

2. The plates were sealed and incubated at 37°C for 2 h.
3. A volume of 150 μL stop buffer, was added into each well of the 96-well plates and the plates were sealed. Addition of 50 m*M* ATP and 0.1% Triton-X in the stop buffer helped reduce nonspecific binding of [γ-^{33}P]ATP to the beads. The concentrations of glutathione- or streptavidin-coated PVT SPA beads are also indicated in the text or figure legends.
4. After a 30-min incubation at room temperature, the plates were centrifuged at 900*g* for 3 min at room temperature using a Sorvall HERMLE centrifuge and then counted in a 1450 MicroBeta liquid-scintillation counter with a crosstalk correction program. The data were analyzed using Prism (GraphPad, San Diego, CA).

3.3. Fluorescence Resonance Energy Transfer Assays for Tyrosine Kinases

1. All reagents were diluted in the assay buffer. poly(Glu:Tyr)/ATP or poly(Glu:Ala:Tyr)/ATP were combined and added in a black 384-well, opaque-walled microtiter plate (*see* **Note 3**).
2. The assay plate was incubated at room temperature for 60 min after the addition of the tyrosine kinase.
3. The assay plate was further incubated for 30 min after the addition of a buffer (20 m*M* Tris-HCl, pH 7.5, 0.35% BSA, 35 m*M* EDTA, 1 *M* KF) containing streptavidin-XLallophycocyanin (SA-XLAPC) and a europium cryptate or chelate labeled antiphosphotyrosine antibody (PT-66) (*see* **Note 4**).
4. Detection of energy transfer was performed on both Packard Discovery and/or Wallac Victor 2 (*see* **Note 5**).

3.4. Fluorescence Polarization Assays for Serine/Threonine Kinases

3.4.1. Evaluation of Binding of Tracers to Different Antibodies

1. Fluorescently labeled tracers were mixed with a number of antibodies in a 96-well plate with a final volume of 200 μL/well FP buffer 1 and incubated at room temperature for 30–60 min.
2. The plate was read in the Analyst. The wavelength of the excitation filter is 485 nm with a band width of 20 nm; the wavelength of the emission filter is 530 nm with a band width of 25 nm. The integration time is 100–300 ms with one read per well. The Z-height was 3 mm. The excitation polarizer is the static polarizer and the emission polarizer is the dynamic polarizer.
3. The fluorescence polarization in millipolar (mP) was calculated using the following equation:

$$\text{Polarization (mP)} = \frac{\left(I_{||} - I_{||C}\right) - g\left(I_{\perp} - I_{\perp C}\right)}{\left(I_{||} - I_{||C}\right) + g\left(I_{\perp} - I_{\perp C}\right)} \times 1000$$

Where $I_{||}$ and $I_{\perp}$ represent the emission intensities of the tracer with the emission polarization parallel and perpendicular to the excitation polarization, respectively. The emission intensities parallel $(I_{||C})$ and perpendicular $(I_{\perp C})$ to the excitation polarization from a control well containing only antibody in the buffer are subtracted from the corresponding intensities from sample wells. For calculation of the millipolar values of the tracer only, $I_{||C}$ and $I_{\perp C}$ were measured from a well containing only buffer. Introduction of $I_{||C}$ and $I_{\perp C}$ in the calculation of millipolar values minimizes effects of background fluorescence from the antibody and/or buffer on determination of fluorescence polarization values. The g factor multiplying the perpendicular emission intensity is used to compensate for the non-zero polarization of the free tracer. In this study, the g factor was fixed at 0.9 that gives a mP value of about 25–35 in the presence of the fluorescein tracer alone.

3.4.2. A Competitive Fluorescence Polarization Assay for PKC

A competitive FP assay has been developed for measurement of kinase activity of PKC. The enzymatic reactions were carried out in 384-well OptiPlates in a final volume of 50 μL of the PKC buffer. The substrate was RFARKGSLRQKNV.

1. To start the reaction, PKC was added to wells of a 384-well plate that contained the substrate and 100 μM ATP.
2. The plate was incubated at room temperature for 90 min.
3. Subsequently, 20 μL of the FP buffer 2 containing antibody 2B9 and fluorescein-RFARKGS(PO$_4$)LRQKNV was added. The final concentrations of 2B9 and fluorescein-RFARKGS(PO$_4$)LRQKNV in the assay mixtures (70 μL) were 400 pM and 250 pM, respectively, or indicated in the text or figure legends.
4. The plate was incubated at room temperature for 30 min and then read in the Analyst. For all FP assays in this study, the polarization (mP) was calculated using the equation described previously.

3.5. Results and Discussion

3.5.1. Scintillation Proximity Assay (SPA) for Serine/Threonine Kinases

Phosphorylation of GST-Rb152-StrepTag was carried out at 37°C for 2 h in the presence of different concentrations of [γ-^{33}P]ATP. The amount of signal detected in the SPA assay in the presence or absence of Cdk4 is illustrated in **Fig. 1**. Both signal (plus enzyme) and background (minus enzyme) increased with the radioactivity added. However, ratios of signal to noise remained relatively unchanged (approx 3:1) regardless of the amount of radioactivity added. **Figure 2** shows the amount of ^{33}PO$_4$ incorporation as a function of time in the SPA assay using GST-Rb152-StrepTag as a substrate. The phosphorylation

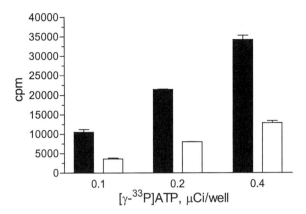

Fig. 1. Phosphorylation of GST-Rb152-StrepTag by Cdk4 with increasing amounts of radioactivity. The reaction was carried out in a final volume of 50 μL Cdk4 buffer at 37°C for 2 h in the presence (closed bars) and absence (open bars) of Cdk4. The concentrations of Cdk4 and GST-Rb152-StrepTag were 40 μg/mL and 390 μg/mL, respectively. The concentration of ATP was 7.5 μM containing different amounts of [γ-^{33}P]ATP (0.1, 0.2, 0.4 (μCi/well) as indicated in the figure. The reactions were terminated by addition of 150 μL of stop buffer per well containing 1.0 mg streptavidin-coated PVT SPA beads. The error bars represent the difference of duplicates in the experiment.

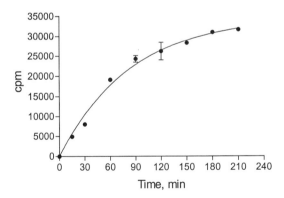

Fig. 2. Time dependence of phosphorylation by Cdk4. The experiment was carried out in a final volume of 50 μL Cdk4 buffer at 37°C. The concentrations of Cdk4 and GST-Rb152-StrepTag were 50 μg/mL and 390 μg/mL, respectively. The concentration of ATP is 7.5 μM (0.2 μCi [γ-^{33}P]ATP/well). The reaction was terminated by addition of 150 μL of stop buffer per well containing 0.5 mg streptavidin-coated PVT SPA beads after an incubation of 15, 30, 60, 90, 120, 150, 180, or 210 min. The error bars represent the difference of duplicates in the experiment. cpm: specific incorporation of radioactivity after background (zero incubation time) subtraction.

Table 1
Comparison of IC$_{50}$ Values Determined in the SPA and Filter-Binding Assay[a]

Compound	SPA (IC$_{50}$, nM)	Filter-binding (IC$_{50}$, nM)
Flavopiridol	220 ± 20	250 ± 50
Compound X	395 ± 15	350 ± 50
Compound Y	195 ± 25	150 ± 25
Compound Z	2250 ± 150	2300 ± 200

[a]The data presented here are mean $\pm$ SEM from at least three independent experiments performed in duplicate. For the SPA assay, the concentration of beads was 0.5 mg/well.

reaction rate was relatively linear up to 90–120 min at 37°C. After 120 min, the incorporation of $^{33}PO_4$ only increased slightly. The ability of several compounds to inhibit Cdk4 kinase activity was evaluated. **Table 1** compares IC$_{50}$ values of four compounds determined in the SPA and filter-binding assay. The IC$_{50}$ values determined in the two assays were comparable.

In conclusion, a high-throughput, homogenous assay for measurement of Cdk4 kinase activity have been successfully developed using the affinity peptide-tagged pRb protein as a substrate. Compared to the published methods, our approach is simple, robust, robotics-friendly, and allows the use of the physiological substrate for screening.

3.5.2. Fluorescence Resonance Energy Transfer Assays for Tyrosine Kinases

An HTR-FRET assay for a tyrosine kinase has been developed using europium-cryptate-labeled antiphoshpotyrosine antibody, PT66. The parameters that have been optimized during the assay development were the concentrations of biotin-polymers, europium-labeled PT66, streptavidin-APC, and kinase. After the assay optimization, we have obtained a signal-to-background ratio of 10:1 (data not shown). We have next compared two polymers as substrates in this FRET assay. These two polymers were biotin-poly (Glu:Ala:Tyr) and biotin-poly (Glu:Tyr). Both polymers have been used as generic substrates in the development of many tyrosine kinases assays by different researchers *(2,3)*. We have found that poly (Glu:Ala:Tyr) was a much more efficient substrate in the tyrosine kinase FRET assay than poly (Glu:Tyr) (**Fig. 3**). Since both of them are random polymers, it is unclear why significantly high phosphorylation was observed at the same concentration of the tyrosine kinase when the poly (Glu:Ala:Tyr) was employed as the substrate. Profiling of FRET

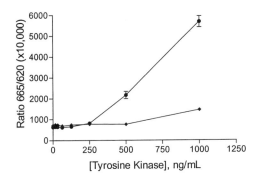

Fig. 3. Phosphorylation of poly (Glu:Ala:Tyr) (●) and poly (Glu:Tyr) (◆) by a tyrosine kinase. The reactions were carried out in 384-well plates with an assay volume of 50 μL at room temperature for 60 min. The concentrations of reagents are: poly(Glu:Ala:Tyr) = 62.5 nM; poly(Glu:Tyr) = 62.5 nM; ATP = 8 μM; SA-APC = 31 nM; Eu-PT66 = 0.8 nM. The concentration of the tyrosine kinase is indicated in the figure.

reagents from various sources with different labeling techniques was shown in **Fig. 4** (*see also* **Note 3**).

3.5.3. Fluorescence Polarization Assays for Serine/Threonine Kinases

3.5.3.1. SELECTION OF ANTIBODIES AND TRACERS

Seven commercially available antiphosphoserine antibodies from different sources have been evaluated. These antibodies fall into two groups. Group 1 includes Biomeda monoclonal antibody (mAb), Biomeda pAb, Sigma, DRI, HTI products, and NEB antibodies. Based on the data from the manufacturers/distributors, antibodies in Group 1 have been proven to bind to the phosphoserine residue in a protein or peptide in either Western blots or enzyme-linked immunosorbent assay (ELISA) assays. Group 2 has only one mAb, 2B9, which reportedly binds to a specific phosphoserine-containing peptide (RFARKGS(PO$_4$)LRQKNV) in an ELISA assay. The antibodies in Group 1 were evaluated in the FP assay against Tracer A, fluorescein-Ahx-TSS(PO$_4$)FAEG and fluorescein (**Fig. 5A**). The background fluorescence polarization was determined in the presence of Tracer A or fluorescein alone. For all antibodies, the difference of fluorescence polarization (mP) between wells containing the antibody plus the tracer and tracer alone ranged from 3–28 mP except polyclonal antibody (pAb) from Biomeda. The difference in fluorescence polarization (mP) between wells containing Biomeda-pAb plus the tracer and tracer alone was 45 mP. However, this antibody turned out to bind to fluorescein instead of the phosphoserine.

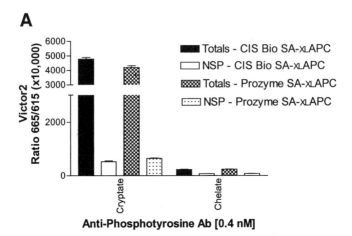

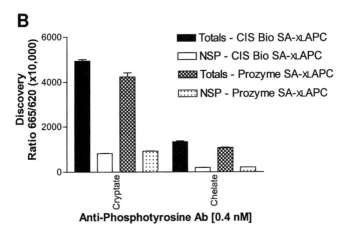

Fig. 4. Reagent profiling in a tyrosine kinase FRET assay. The reactions were performed in 384-well plates. Poly (Glu:Ala:Tyr) (31 nM) was used as substrate. The concentration of kinase and ATP was 1 µg/mL and 8 µM, respectively. (**A**) the plate was read on Victor 2; (**B**) the same plate was read on Discovery.

We next evaluated 2B9, a phosphopeptide-specific antibody, against three tracers: Tracer A = fluorescein-Ahx-TSS(PO₄)FAEG; Tracer B = fluorescein-GS(PO₄)FAEG; Tracer C = fluorescein-RFARKGS(PO₄)LRQKNV (**Fig. 5B**). This mAb showed significant binding to Tracer C only. The difference in polarization (mP) between wells containing 2B9 plus Tracer C and Tracer C alone was approx 160 mP. This antibody did not bind to fluorescein. The antibodies in Group 1 did not show significant binding to either Tracer C or B (data not shown). The titration of 2B9 is shown in **Fig. 6**. The polarization signal in mP increased with the concentration of 2B9 and then reached a plateau. 2B9 rec-

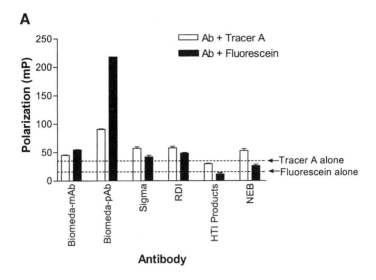

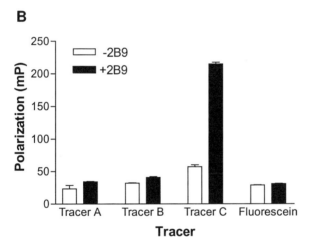

Fig. 5. **(A)** Selection of antiphosphoserine antibodies: The assays were carried out in 96-well plates with a final volume of 200 µL FP buffer 1. Tracer A was fluorescein-Ahx-TSS(PO₄)FAEG at 2 nM. Fluorescein dye was 2 nM. The concentrations of antibodies were as follows: Biomeda-mAb = 13 µg/mL; Biomeda-pAb = 1:50 dilution; Sigma = 106 µg/mL; RDI = 106 µg/mL; HTI products = 66 µg/mL; NEB = 1:50 dilution; 2B9 = 125 ng/mL. The dashed lines (Tracer A alone and fluorescein alone) in the figure indicate polarization values in the absence of any antibody. The error bars represent the difference of duplicates in the experiment. **(B)** Selection of tracers: The assays were carried out in 96-well plates with a final volume of 200 µL FP buffer 1. 2B9 was added to wells containing different tracers. The concentration of 2B9 was 125 ng/mL. Three tracers were evaluated: Tracer A = fluorescein-Ahx-TSS(PO₄)FAEG; Tracer B = fluorescein-GS(PO₄)FAEG; Tracer C = fluorescein-RFARKGS(PO₄)LRQKNV. Fluorescein dye was used as a control. The concentration of all three tracers and fluorescein was 2 nM. The error bars represent the difference of duplicates in the experiment.

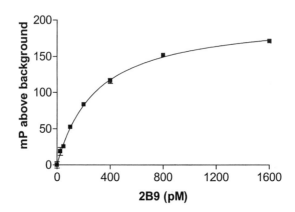

Fig. 6. Titration of monoclonal antiphosphoserine antibody, 2B9. The experiment was carried out in a 96-well plate with a final assay volume of 200 µL. Fluorescein-RFARKGS(PO₄)LRQKNV (250 p*M*) was mixed with different concentrations of 2B9 as indicated in the figure. The error bars represent the difference of duplicates in the experiment.

ognizes a specific phosphopeptide sequence, RFARKGS (PO₄)LRQKNV, and is originally used in an ELISA assay by Medical and Biological Laboratory, Inc. In fact, all antibodies we tested above are reported to work in either Western blots or ELISA assays by their manufacturers or distributors, suggesting that FP assays require higher affinity antibodies than other assays. This is consistent with the data obtained from the tyrosine kinase FP assay. Indeed, our data indicate that 2B9 has very high affinity to fluorescein-RFARKGS(PO₄)LR QKNV (K_d = 250 ± 34 p*M*).

3.5.3.2. A Competitive Fluorescence Polarization Assay for PKC

In order to develop a robust FP assay for PKC, a competitive approach was employed. In the competitive FP assay, unlabeled peptide, RFARKGSLRQKNV was used as a substrate in the enzymatic reactions in black 384-well plates. After phosphorylation, 2B9 and fluorescent tracer, fluorescein-RFARK GS(PO₄)LRQKNV was added to wells in the plate. Unlabeled phosphopeptide competes with the tracer for 2B9, resulting in a decrease in polarization. In the presence of PKC, the polarization in mP decreased with an increase in the substrate concentration and reached a plateau at the substrate concentration of greater than 0.3 µ*M*. In the absence of PKC, the polarization in mP remained constant over the substrate concentration up to 2 µ*M*. The maximum change in polarization between plus and minus PKC was approx 100 mP.

We have determined the IC_{50} value of a known inhibitor, staurosporine, of PKC in the FP assay. The polarization signal increased with the concentration

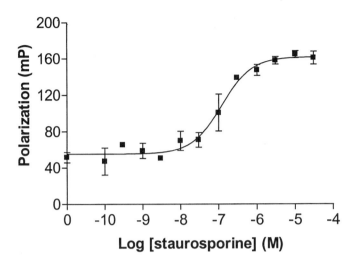

Fig. 7. Inhibition of the PKC kinase activity by staurosporine. The phosphorylation reactions were carried out in 384-well plates with a volume of 50 μL reaction buffer in presence of different concentrations of staurosporine as indicated in the figure. The concentration of the peptide substrate and PKC was 1 μM and 27 ng/mL, respectively. The concentration of phosphatidylserine was 50 μg/mL. The error bars represent the difference of duplicates in the experiment.

of staurosporine since it is a competitive FP assay. **Figure 7** shows a representative inhibition curve of PKC. The IC_{50} value of staurosporine for PKC was 720 ± 160 nM (mean $\pm$ SEM, $n = 6$).

As we indicated above, 2B9 binds to the specific phosphopeptide sequence, RFARKGS (PO$_4$)LRQKNV. The next question we have asked was whether a generic or semigeneric FP assay can be developed using this antibody. Our recent data indicate that 2B9 can be used to develop a semi-generic FP assay in 384- and/or 1536-well plates for serine/threonine kinases such as PKA, casein kinase-1, and calmodulin dependent kinase-2 (manuscript in preparation).

3.6. Comparisons

There are many different technologies for the development of HTS assays for discovering kinase inhibitors. Different technologies may have different sensitivity, dynamic range, and signal-to-background ratio for developing an assay for a specific kinase. Furthermore, different sets of hits may be discovered by different technologies. Therefore, it is important to compare these technologies during the assay development and select an appropriate technology for HTS of a specific kinase target. In this section, I have compared and contrasted SPA, FRET, and FP for the development of kinase assays.

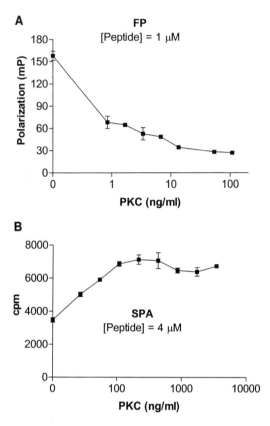

Fig. 8. Comparison of FP and SPA assays for serine/threonine kinase, PKC. (A) The FP assay was carried out in a 384-well plate with a volume of 50 μL PKC buffer. The concentration of the peptide substrate (RFARKGSLRQKNV) was 1 μM. PKC was titrated. (B) The SPA was carried out in a 384-well plate with a volume of 50 μL PKC buffer in the presence of 4 μM biotinylated peptide (biotin-RFARKGS LRQKNV). The concentrations of PKC are illustrated in the figure. [γ-^{33}P]ATP was 400,000 cpm/well. After 2-h incubation at room temperature, 30 μL stop buffer with 1 mg streptavidin-coated PVT SPA beads was added to each well. The plate was incubated at room temperature for 30 min and centrifuged. The radioactivity was measured in a TriLux plate reader. The error bars represent the difference of duplicates in the experiments.

3.6.1. Comparison of SPA and FP for Serine/Threonine Kinases

The sensitivity of FP and SPA was compared in the development of PKC kinase assays in terms of the amount of the kinase required to yield a similar signal (**Fig. 8**). Both FP and SPA assays were carried out in 384-well plates with a final assay volume of 50 μL PKC buffer containing 50 μg/mL phosphatidylserine. In the competitive FP assay, the peptide substrate, RFARKGSLRQKNV, was 1 μM. PKC was titrated. The polarization in mP decreased with an increase in the PKC concentration and then reached a plateau at the PKC concentration of 10 ng/mL. In comparison, there was no significant phosphorylation detected in the SPA assay when the concentrations of the substrate (biotin-RFARKGSLRQKNV) and PKC were 4 μM and 10 ng/mL. A signal-to-background ratio of 2:1 was observed in the SPA assay when the concentration of PKC was 220 ng/mL. These data indicate that for generating a reasonable signal, less PKC and peptide substrate were required in the FP assay than in the SPA assay.

3.6.2. Comparison of SPA, FRET, and FP for Tyrosine Kinases

We have compared SPA, FRET, and FP for a tyrosine kinase (TK) in terms of sensitivity and dose-response curves of a nonspecific kinase inhibitor, staurosporine (**Fig. 9**). The results indicate that for the development of a robust assay for the tyrosine kinase in 384-well format, SPA required 200 ng/well kinase; FRET required 1 ng/well kinase; FP required 4 ng/well kinase. We next examined the inhibition of the tyrosine kinase activity by staurosporine in all assay formats. Our data indicate that $IC_{50}s$ determined in all three assays are consistent. Therefore, FRET and FP may be chosen for this tyrosine kinase for the reason that they require less kinase. However, our recent data suggest that different sets of hits were discovered after screening a large number of compounds using these different assay technologies (data not shown). We don't know yet which assay technology would discover more physiologically relevant hit compounds since biologically relevant assays (e.g., cell-based assays) for those hits have not been developed.

4. Notes

1. In our first attempts to establish a high-throughput, homogeneous SPA assay for Cdk4 using the natural protein substrate, GST-Rb152 was employed as the substrate and GST was used as the detection tag. After the phosphorylation reaction was completed, glutathione-coated SPA beads, in increasing concentrations, were added to the reaction mixture. The radioactivity profiles detected with increasing concentrations of glutathione-coated SPA beads were almost identical in the presence or absence of GST-Rb152. Since significant phosphorylation of GST-Rb152 by Cdk4 was seen in the filtration assay (data not shown), failure to detect specific phosphorylation in SPA may be due to a weak interaction between GST and the glutathione-coated SPA beads as well as to the amount of glutathione coupled to PVT SPA beads.

2. Since phosphorylation of GST-Rb152 was not detected in the SPA assay using glutathione-coated beads, we investigated other tags in order to develop an SPA. A nine amino acid peptide (AWRHPQFGG), named StrepTag (*18*), which dis-

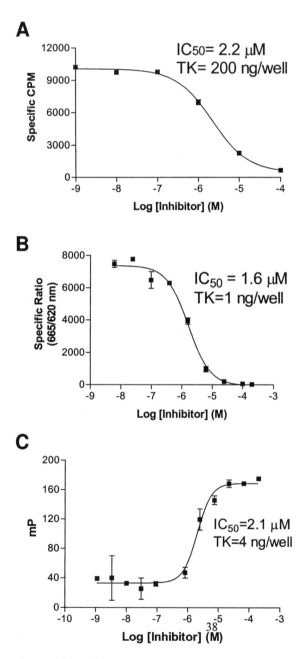

Fig. 9. Comparison of SPA (**A**), FRET (**B**) and FP (**C**) assays for a tyrosine kinase. The phosphorylation reactions were carried out in a 384-well plate with a volume of 50 μL. Poly (Glu:Ala:Tyr) (31 n*M*) was used as a substrate. The inhibitor, staurosporine, was titrated as indicated in the figure. The concentration of the tyrosine kinase and the IC_{50} values of staurosporine were also indicated in the figure.

plays intrinsic binding affinity to streptavidin, was chosen as the alternative. We have therefore constructed a StrepTag at the C-terminus of the GST-Rb512, using recombinant DNA technology. The gene construct and the expressed protein (GST-Rb152-StrepTag) proved to be critical for the development of a high-throughput, homogeneous assay for Cdk4.

3. The effect of reagents from different sources on the development of the FRET assay for the tyrosine kinase was studied (**Fig. 4**). PT66 labeled with europium cryptate or europium chelate was compared in the tyrosine kinase FRET assay. SA-APC from either CIS bio International or Prozyme was also compared. After the tyrosine kinase FRET assay was completed, the plates were read in either Discovery (Packard Instrument, Meriden, CT) or Victor 2 (PerkinElmer Wallac). The data indicated that the FRET signals (Totals) generated in the assay with europium cryptate-labeled PT66 from Packard Instrument were greater than those generated with europium chelate-labeled PT66 from PerkinElmer Wallac. However, there was no significant difference in signal-to-background ratios (Totals vs NSP) between using either europium cryptate or chelate-labeled PT66. There was also no significant difference in signals (Totals) between using SA-APC from either CIS bio International (France) or Prozyme (Dan Leandro, CA).

4. The results suggest that the robust FRET assays for tyrosine kinases can be developed using reagents with different labeling techniques.

5. Signal profiling of reagents was similar when the plates were read on either Discovery or Victor 2. Therefore, both Discover and Victor 2 can be used for reliably detecting FRET signals in tyrosine kinase assays

Acknowledgments

I want to thank Dr. Matthew Sills and Dr. Robert Schweitzer at Novartis Institute for Biomedical Research for their intellectual support. I want to thank Donna Yarwood, Quynhchi Pham, and Michael Chin at Novartis Institute for Biomedical Research for their excellent technical support. Finally, I would like to thank Dr. Bhabatosh Chaudhuri at Novartis Pharma AG, Basel, Switzerland for providing Cdk4 kinase and substrate.

References

1. Beveridge, M., Park Y. W., Hermes, J., Marenghi, A., Brophy, and G., Santos, A. (2000) Detection of p56(lck) kinase activity using scintillation proximity assay in 384-well format and imaging proximity assay in 384- and 1536-well format. *J. Biomol. Screen* **5,** 205–212.

2. Braunwalder, A. F., Yarwood, D. R, Sills, M. A., and Lipson, K. E. (1996a) Measurement of the protein tyrosine kinase activity of c-src using time-resolved fluorometry of europium chelates. *Anal. Biochem.* **238,** 159–164.

3. Braunwalder, A. F., Yarwood, D. R., Hall, T., Missbach, M., Lipson, K. E., and Sills, M. A. (1996b) A solid-phase assay for the determination of protein tyrosine kinase activity of c-src using scintillating microtitration plates. *Anal. Biochem.* **234,** 23–26.

4. Hemmila, I. (1999) LANCEtrade mark: homogeneous assay platform for HTS. *J. Biomol. Screen.* **4**, 303–308.
5. Parker, G. J., Law, T. L., Lenoch, F. J., and Bolger, R. E. (2000) Development of high throughput screening assays using fluorescence polarization: nuclear receptor-ligand-binding and kinase/phosphatase assays. *J. Biomol. Screen.* **5**, 77–88.
6. Wouters, F. S. and Bastiaens, P. (1999) Fluorescence lifetime imaging of receptor tyrosine kinase activity in cell. *Curr. Biol.* **9**, 1127–1130.
7. Wu, J. J., Yarwood, D. R., Chaudhuri, B., Muller, L., Zurini, M., and Sills, M. A. (2000) Measurement of Cdk4 kinase activity using an affinity peptide-tagging technology. *Comb. Chem. High Throughput Screen* **3**, 27–36.
8. Wu, J. J., Yarwood, D. R., Pham, Q., and Sills, M. A. (2000) Identification of a high affinity anti-phosphoserine antibody for the development of a homogeneous fluorescence polarization assay of Protein Kinase C. *J. Biomol. Screening* **5**, 23–30.
9. Kowski. T. J. and Wu, J. J. (2000) Fluorescence polarization is a useful technology for reagent reduction in assay miniaturization. *Comb. Chem. High Throughput Screen* **3**, 437–444.
10. Fowler, A., Swift, D., Hemsley, P., et al. (2000) A 1536 well fluorescence polarization assay for the Ser/Thr kinase JNK-1, Abstract, the Society for Biomolecular Screening 6th Annual Conference and Exhibition, pp. 196.
11. Storch, E., Ragan, S., Born, T., Chipman, S., and Wu, J. J. (2000) Evaluation of different microtiter plate readers for the development of FP and HTR-FRET assays in 384- and 1536-well plates. Abstract for the Society for Biomolecular Screening 6th Annual Conference and Exhibition, pp. 246.
12. Brophy, G., Blair, J., and Pither, R. (1995) p34^{cdc2} kinase activity determination using the scintillation proximity assay (SPA). *Abstract for the 9th International Conference on Second Messengers and Phosphoproteins.* Nashville, TN. pp. 274.
13. Gobel, J., Saussy, D. L., and Goetz, A. S. (1999) Development of scintillation-proximity assays for alpha adrenoceptors. *J. Pharmacol. Toxicol. Methods* **42**, 237–244.
14. Liu, J., Feldman, P. A., Lippy, J. S., Bobkova, E., Kurilla, M. G., and Chung, T. D. (2001) A scintillation proximity assay for RNA detection. *Anal. Biochem.* **289**, 239–245.
15. Sherr, C. J. (1996) Cancer cell cycles. *Science* **274**, 1672–1677.
16. Matsushime, H., Quelle, D. E., Shurtleff, S. A., Shibuya, M., Sherr, C. J., and Kato, J. Y. (1994) D-type cyclin-dependent kinase activity in mammalian cells. *Mol. Cell. Biol.* **14**, 2066–2076.
17. Kitagawa, M., Higashi, H., Jung, H. K., Suzuki-Takahashi, I., Ikeda, M., Tamai, K., et al. (1996) The consensus motif for phosphorylation by cyclin D1-Cdk4 is different from that for phosphorylation by cyclin A/E-Cdk2. *EMBO J.* **15**, 7060–7069.
18. Schmidt, T. G. and Skerra, A. (1993) The random peptide library-assisted engineering of a C-terminal affinity peptide, useful for the detection and purification of a functional Ig Fv fragment. *Protein Eng.* **6**, 109–122.
19. Stenroos, K., Hurskainen, P., Eriksson, S., Hemmila, I., Blomberg, K., and Lindqvist, C. (1998) Homogeneous time-resolved IL-2-IL-2R alpha assay using fluorescence resonance energy transfer. *Cytokine* **10**, 495–499.

20. Lynch, A. B., Loiacono, K. A., Tiong, C. L., Adams, S. E., and MacNeil, I. A. (1997) A fluorescence polarization based Src-SH2 binding assay. *Anal. Biochem.* **247,** 77–82.
21. Wu, P., Brasseur, M., and Schindler, U. (1997) A high-throughput STAT binding assay using fluorescence polarization. *Anal. Biochem.* **249,** 29–36.
22. Meijer, L., Borgne, A., Mulner, O., Chong, J. P., Blow, J., Inagaki, N., et al. (1997) Biochemical and cellular effects of roscovitine, a potent and selective inhibitor of the cyclin-dependent kinases cdc2, cdk2 and cdk5. *Eur. J. Biochem.* **243,** 527–536.
23. Phelps, D. E. and Xiong, Y. (1997) Assay for activity of mammalian cyclin D-dependent kinases CDK4 and CDK6. *Methods Enzymol.* **283,** 194–205.

5

Electrochemiluminescence

A Technology Evaluation and Assay Reformatting of the Stat6/P578 Protein–Peptide Interaction

Robert H. Schweitzer and Laura Abriola

1. Introduction

Biochemical assays used in high-throughput screening (HTS) to identify lead compounds in drug discovery have been formatted using a wide variety of detection techniques. These include radiometric, colorimetric, fluorescent, and enzyme-linked immunosorbent assays (ELISA). Each technique has its strengths and weaknesses. Radiometric assays can be made homogeneous, with no separation steps requiring washing or filtration. Such techniques include scintillation proximity assay (SPA, Amersham Pharmacia Biotech), where the scintillant is contained in a bead, and ScintiPlates® (Perkin-Elmer Wallac) or FlashPlates® (NEN), where the scintillant is contained in the microtiter plate itself. These radiometric techniques are well established, with a wide variety of assays available from many different vendors. Two drawbacks to radiometric assays are the signal-to-background ratio of these assays is typically less than other techniques and the use of radioactive materials are hazardous to the scientist and the environment. When feasible, colorimetric assays are generally easy to format and to run, though often they do not have a very broad dynamic range, since absorbance can typically only be accurately measured in a narrow range (0.1–1.5 OD). Fluorescent techniques offer a wider dynamic range, and are often very sensitive, making it possible to measure low-analyte concentrations. Even so, some compound libraries contain fluorescent compounds, which can interfere with the fluorescence of the label, resulting in false-negatives

From: *Methods in Molecular Biology, vol. 190: High Throughput Screening: Methods and Protocols*
Edited by: W. P. Janzen © Humana Press Inc., Totowa, NJ

or -positives depending on the assay format. This problem can partially be avoided by using time-gated detection, since in many though not all cases, the compound fluorescence is short-lived compared with that of some labels. Techniques such as ELISA and the dissociation-enhanced lanthanide fluoroimmunoassay (DELFIA®, Wallac) are also very well-established and have a wide dynamic range. However, they can be very time-consuming, because many wash steps must be used in the assays. With the ever-increasing compound library sizes used in drug discovery, time-consuming assays are undesirable.

Researchers in the pharmaceutical industry are continually searching for new ways of constituting biochemical assays. They seek to improve sensitivity, reliability, and safety while reducing costs and timelines. Before purchasing a new technology, it is important to carry out a thorough evaluation to assess the reliability and sensitivity of the assay biochemistry and instrumentation. A good understanding of the scientific principles of the technique is important in the evaluation. Each HTS laboratory has its particular requirements, and experience gained during the evaluation can be used to implement successful technologies more efficiently.

1.1. Electrochemiluminescence

A series of experiments were conducted to determine the applicability of electrochemiluminescence (ECL) to HTS. ECL offers many potential advantages. The assays are easy to develop, have a wide dynamic range, and are very sensitive. Also, the assays are essentially homogeneous from the operator's point of view. The wash step takes place within the detection cell after the aspiration of the well contents. The use of ECL in a wide variety of assays is well established, including the detection of biomolecules *(1–5)*, cells *(6)*, bacterial spores *(7)*, toxins *(8)*, enzyme activities *(9,10)*, protein-peptide interactions *(11)*, and polymerase chain reaction (PCR) products *(12–15)*, as wells as determination of binding constants *(16)* and cellular responses *(17–20)*.

Assays formatted for ECL use a ruthenium chelate label and a magnetic bead (**Fig. 1**). The assay is set up so that the amount of ruthenium that is bound to the bead reflects the level of the biological activity that is being measured. Practically, this means that one component of the assay needs to be bound to the bead and another component needs to be labeled with ruthenium *(21,22)*. Which component is bound to the bead and which is labeled with ruthenium depends on the reagents used. For example, biotinylated reagents can be captured using streptavidin-coated beads or labeled using ruthenated streptavidin, while membranes are generally only captured on wheat-germ agglutinin (WGA) or polylysine coated beads.

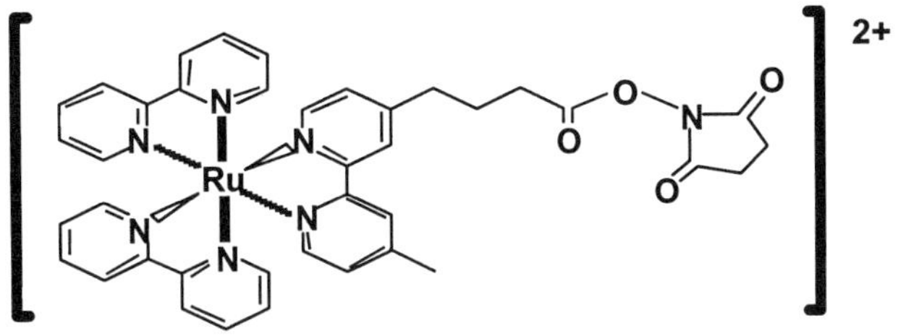

Fig. 1. The tris-bipyridine NHS-ester ruthenium complex used to label antibodies and other proteins for ECL.

Table 1
A List of Ruthenium-Chelate Labeling Chemistries, and Their Labeling Groups or Molecules

Conjugate functional group	Used to label
NHS ester	Primary amines
Maleimide	Thiols
Amine	Carboxyls
Hydrazide	Carbohydrates
Phosphoramidite	Oligonucleotides

There are five ruthenium conjugates available from IGEN with different chemically active groups to be used for attaching the ruthenium chelate to biological reagents: NHS ester, hydrazide, amine, maleimide, and phosphoramidite (**Table 1**). For the work shown in this chapter, the tris-bipyridine-NHS ester was used to label different antibodies. The labeling procedure for antibodies is quite simple, and can be carried out in a few hours.

Several methods can be used to attach biomolecules to the magnetic beads. The most common choice is the streptavidin-biotin interaction. If a biotinylated reagent is available for the assay in question, then the streptavidin-coated magnetic beads provide a simple method to capture the assay. Other magnetic beads are also available from IGEN, including beads with antibodies to a specific assay reagent; WGA and polylysine beads for picking up membranes; and Ni-NTA beads used to bind 6-His-labeled proteins. IGEN obtains their beads from Dynal, and other types of beads are available from this company. The beads are typically 2.8 μm in diameter.

The ECL-detection cell consists of a magnet, which attracts the beads to the electrode, a window through which a light signal passes, and a photodiode for detecting the luminescence (**Fig. 2**). Once assay incubation is complete, the beads are aspirated into the detection cell. Although the assay is "homogeneous" from the operator's point of view, in that only reagent additions are necessary, there is a wash step that occurs in the detection cell. After the beads are captured, the assay buffer is washed away and replaced with IGEN's Origen assay buffer containing tripropylamine (TPA). The ECL signal is generated by redox reactions at the electrode, and is proportional to the amount of ruthenium that is captured on the beads. Only the ruthenium chelate that is within the diffusion layer of the electrode contributes to the signal, reducing the contribution of potentially interfering signals in the bulk sample. This, coupled with the wash step within the detection cell, provides for a wide dynamic range and high sensitivity.

The ECL signal is generated by a series of redox reactions (**Fig. 3**). The Ru^{2+}-chelate complex is oxidized at the electrode to create a Ru^{3+} complex. TPA is also oxidized at the electrode to form a positive radical, which then deprotenates to form a neutral radical. This neutral radical then reduces the Ru^{3+} complex to create a divalent excited-state, Ru^{*2+} complex. As this excited state relaxes it emits a photon, which is detected by the photodiode. The Ru^{2+} complex can then be reoxidized, and the cycle is repeated. In this way, the ECL signal is catalytic in the Ru^{2+} chelate complex. Several photons can be generated from one label, contributing to the high sensitivity of the technique. Because the TPA consumed in the reaction is present in large excess it does not limit the assay's sensitivity. Once the ECL signal is measured, the magnet is turned off and the beads are released and washed away. The detection cell is flushed with a cleaning solution followed by the Origen assay buffer. The instrument is now ready to aspirate from the next well.

This paper presents the conversion and optimization for HTS of a protein-peptide interaction assay, Stat6/P578. Additional examples of a protein-protein interaction assay, Myc/Max, and a Ser/Thr kinase assay, Cdk4, will also be discussed. These assays were chosen because they had been previously developed in alternative HTS formats, which provided a good basis for comparison. Much of the process of adapting these assays to ECL would be the same when considering other assay technologies, particularly bead-based ones.

1.2. Optimization Process

The process used to optimize the assays described here is one that is often used in HTS, though it is not the only process that may be used. Its advantages are ease of use, both conceptually and operationally, and the results are very often adequate for the needs of the assay. However, the parameters being opti-

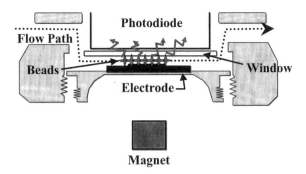

Fig. 2. The IGEN ECL flow cell. The beads are captured on the electrode with a magnet, the buffer is exchanged, the magnet is released, and a series of redox reactions at the electrode result in light detected by a photodiode. This ECL signal is proportional to the amount of ruthenium bound to the magnetic beads.

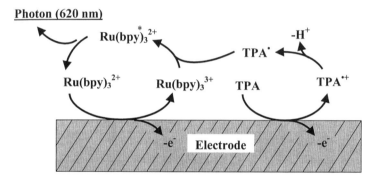

Fig. 3. Tris-bipyridine Ru^{2+} ($Ru(bpy)_3^{2+}$) and tripropylamine (TPA) are oxidized at the electrode. After deprotenating the neutral TPA radical reduces the oxidized ruthenium resulting in an excited state Ru^{*2+} complex. As this excited state relaxes, it emits a photon at 620 nm, which is detected by a photodiode.

mized in the assay are likely to be dependent on each other. Better conditions may be found, if one were to use an experimental-design strategy that samples parameter space more thoroughly than is possible with simple concentration titrations. Experimental design programs that facilitate a more complete exploration of parameter space have been available for some time, though the complexity of the reagent manipulations have limited their use in some HTS laboratories. Fortunately, experimental design programs that are coupled to an automated pipetting device are now being marketed (e.g., by Beckman-Coulter Sagian) and should allow a wider use of experimental design programs for assay optimization.

1.3. Data Analysis

The validity of an assay for HTS depends on the ability to see meaningful changes in signal due to the effect of a compound. A combination of two factors is important in determining whether the changes seen in an assay are meaningful: the signal-to-background ratio or signal window, and the standard deviations of the background and of the uninhibited signals. For assays that have a very low standard deviation (SD) a signal window as small as 2:1 may be meaningful. However, assays that have a high variability would require a much greater signal-to-background ratio in order for the change in signal to be interpreted as due to the compound and not due to the inherent variations of the assay. A measure of the quality of an assay is the Z' factor *(24)*, where

$$Z' = \frac{\left(3\sigma_{C+} + 3\sigma_{C-}\right)}{\left|\mu_{c+} - \mu_{c-}\right|}$$

and $\sigma_{c\pm}$ are the standard deviations and $\mu_{c\pm}$ are the mean of the positive and negative controls. An assay with a Z' between 0.5 and 1.0 is considered to be an excellent assay for HTS, while values lower than 0.5 would indicate that the assay is less well-suited for HTS. Experiments were generally performed in triplicate on the microtiter plate, and the average was used for analysis.

The dose-response curves were fit to a sigmoidal dose-response function with a variable slope:

$$Signal = \frac{S_{max} - S_{min}}{1 + 10^{(\log I_o - x)p}} + S_{min}$$

where S_{max} and S_{min} are the maximum and minimum signal levels, I_o is the 50% inhibition concentration, x is the concentration of the inhibitor for each data point, and p is the Hill coefficient.

1.4. ECL Instrumentation

All experiments were performed in 96-well microtiter plates, and brought to a final volume of 300 μL. The well contents were transferred with a Pasteur pipet to 12 × 75-mm test tubes, which were placed in the IGEN Origen single-channel instrument. Some of the variability in the results shown here may be due to this transfer step. The single-channel Origen maintains the magnetic beads in suspension by vortexing the test tubes prior to aspirating the contents of each tube into the detection cell to be read. A maximum of 50 tubes may be loaded on the instrument at a time. Each tube is read in a little over 1 min. The large assay volumes chosen were dictated by the minimum final volume of 300 μL necessary for detection with the test tube-based instrument. Some experiments were also done in volumes as low as 50 μL, and brought to a final volume of 300 μL by addition of the magnetic-bead suspension. Recently, we have run experiments with the M-series eight-channel Origen. It aspirates directly from an entire column of a 96-well microtiter plate, then reads the contents simultaneously. These recent experiments were performed in 150 μL final volume in polypropylene round-bottom plates.

2. Materials

2.1. Original DELFIA Stat5/P578 Interaction Assay

2.1.1. Anti-Stat6 Antibody Labeling

1. Europium-labeling buffer: 50 mM NaHCO$_3$, pH 8.5, 150 mM NaCl.
2. Anti-Stat6 antibody, S-20 (Santa Cruz Biotechnology, Cat. no. Sc-621x).
3. Elution buffer: 50 mM NaHCO$_3$, pH 8.5, 150 mM NaCl, 0.05% NaN$_3$.
4. Stock BSA, 10% in deionized water.
5. Sephadex G-50 (Sigma).
6. 1.5 × 30 cm econo-column, Bio-Rad, Cat. no. 737-1532).

2.1.2. Coating Plates

1. Streptavidin plate coating solution: 8 mM Na$_2$CO$_3$, 17 mM NaHCO$_3$, pH 9.6, 500 mM NaCl, 10 μg/mL streptavidin.
2. DELFIA wash buffer: 10 mM Tris-HCl, pH 8.0, 150 mM NaCl, 0.1% Casein, 0.2% Tween-20.
3. Assay buffer: 10 mM Tris-HCl, pH 8.0, 150 mM NaCl, 0.1% Casein.
4. b-P578: Biotinylated 15-mer phosphopeptide, biotin-GPPGEAGy*KAFSSLL, Neosystem (France) or Cambridge Research Biochemicals (UK).

2.1.3. DELFIA Screening Assay

1. Europium labeled anti-Stat6 antibody (*see* **Subheading 3.1.1.** for labeling details).
2. Stat6: Signal transducer and activator of transcription 6 (Stat6) was produced as a C-terminus 6-His-tagged protein and purified by Graham et al. *(23)* with nickel and phosphotyrosine affinity columns to approx 95% purity.
3. Assay buffer: 10 mM Tris-HCl, pH 8.0, 150 mM NaCl, 0.1% Casein.
4. DELFIA enhancement solution (Perkin-Elmer Wallac, Cat. no. B118-100).
5. FluoroNunc Maxisorp microplates (Fisher, Cat. no. 12-565-290C).
6. The Wallac Victor™ (1420) (Perkin-Elmer Wallac Inc., Gaithersburg, MD).

2.2. Labeling Antibodies with Ruthenium

1. Anti-Stat6 antibody, S-20 (Santa Cruz Biotechnology, Cat. no. Sc-621x).
2. Anti-phospho-retinoblastoma tumor-suppressor protein Ser795 antibody (New England Biolabs, Cat. no. 9301B).
3. Anti-GST antibody (Amersham Pharmacia Biotech, Cat. no. 27-4577).
4. PBS: 8 mM sodium phosphate, 2 mM potassium phosphate, pH 7.4, 140 mM sodium chloride.

5. DMSO: Dimethylsulfoxide (Sigma).
6. NHS-ester ruthenium labeling reagent (IGEN International, Cat. no. 402-001-01).
7. 2 *M* Glycine solution, Sigma.
8. Protein concentration kit (Pierce, Micro BCA, Cat. no. 23231).
9. Spin-filtration system (Millipore Centricon, YM-30).
10. Sephadex G-25 column (Amersham Pharmacia Biotech NAP5, Cat. no. 17-0853-01).

2.3. ECL Stat6/P578 Interaction Assay

2.3.1. Assay Optimization (Materials List is the Same for All Other Sections)

1. Ruthenium labeled anti-Stat6 antibody (*see* **Subheading 3.2.**).
2. Stat6: Signal transducer and activator of transcription 6 (Stat6) was produced as a C-terminus 6-His-tagged protein and purified by Graham et al. *(23)* with nickel and phosphotyrosine affinity columns to approx 95% purity.
3. b-P578: Biotinylated 15-mer phosphopeptide, biotin-GPPGEAGy*KAFSSLL, Neosystem (France) or Cambridge Research Biochemicals (UK).
4. P578: Non-biotinylated 15-mer phosphopeptide, GPPGEAGy*KAFSSLL, Neosystem (France) or Cambridge Research Biochemicals (UK).
5. ECL Stat6/P578 interaction assay buffer: 10 m*M* Tris-HCL, pH 8.0, 150 m*M* NaCl, and a bead-blocking component either, casein, BSA from Sigma, or Pierce Superblock as indicated in the text.
6. Streptavidin-coated magnetic beads (IGEN International, Cat. no. 401-175-01).
7. Ninety-six-well microtiter plates (Corning Costar, Cat. no. 3915 and Cat. no. 9670).
8. ORIGEN, or an Eight-channel M-series ORIGEN (IGEN International).

2.4 Additional Assay Conversion Examples

2.4.1 Myc Max

1. 6-His-Max produced in house.
2. GST-Myc produced in house.
3. Biotinylated anti-6-His antibody (Clontech, Cat. no. 8904-1). The biotin labeling is completely analogous to the ruthenium labeling described in **Subheading 3.2.**
4. Ruthenium labeled anti-GST antibody (Amersham Pharmacia Biotech, cat. no. 27-4577). (*See* **Subheading 3.2.** for labeling details).
5. Streptavidin-coated magnetic beads (IGEN International, Cat. no. 401-175-01).
6. Ni-NTA coated magnetic beads (IGEN International).
7. Ninety-six-well microtiter plates (Corning Costar, Cat. no. 3915 and Cat. no. 9670).
8. Biacore 2000 Biosensor (Biacore AB).
9. Biacore sensor chip SA (Cat. no. BR-1000-32).
10. ORIGEN, or an Eight-channel M-series ORIGEN (IGEN International).

2.4.2. Cdk4

1. Buffer conditions as described in Wu et al. *(28)*.
2. Cdk4 produced in house as described in Wu et al. *(28)*.

3. Rb fragment kinase substrate produced in house as described in Wu et al. *(28)*.
4. Ruthenium labeled anti-phospho-retinoblastoma tumor-suppressor protein Ser795 antibody (New England Biolabs, Cat. no. 9301B). (*See* **Subheading 3.2.** for labeling details).
5. Streptavidin-coated magnetic beads (IGEN International, Cat. no. 401-175-01).
6. Ninety-six-well microtiter plates (Corning Costar, Cat. no. 3915 and Cat. no. 9670).
7. ORIGEN, or an Eight-channel M-series ORIGEN (IGEN International).

3. Methods

3.1. Original DELFIA Stat5/P578 Interaction Assay

The Stat6 interaction with a biotinylated phosphopeptide (b-P578) has been previously screened as a DELFIA. The DELFIA assay involved two overnight incubations and four wash steps, where the microtiter plate was washed two or three times at each step.

3.1.1. Anti-Stat6 Antibody Labeling

1. Add europium-labeling buffer to 1 mg of antibody in 1 mL buffer.
2. Incubate overnight at room temperature.
3. Pass solution over a Sephadex G-50 column equilibrated with elution buffer.
4. Add BSA to 0.1%.
5. Aliquot and store at –80°C.

3.1.2. Coating Plates

1. Add 50 µL/well of streptavidin solution, 500 ng/well.
2. Incubate overnight at 4°C.
3. Wash three times with 200 µL/well of DELFIA wash buffer.
4. Add 50 µL/well of b-P578 30 ng/well phosphopeptide in assay buffer.
5. Incubate overnight at 4°C.
6. Wash three times with 200 µL/well of wash buffer.
7. Add 200 µL/well of assay buffer.
8. Incubate 1 h at room temperature.
9. Wash twice with 200 µL/well of wash buffer.
10. Store plates at –20°C, until needed.

3.1.3. DELFIA Screening Assay

1. Add 5 µL/well of test compound (*see* **Notes 4** and **5**).
2. Add 45 µL/well of Stat6 (90 ng/well) and Europium labeled anti-Stat6 antibody (1–4 ng/well).
3. Incubate 1 h at room temperature.
4. Wash three times with 200 µL/well of assay buffer.
5. Add 100 µL/well of DELFIA enhancement solution.
6. Read plates in Perkin-Elmer Wallac Victor.

3.2. Labeling Antibodies with Ruthenium

The NHS-ester ruthenium conjugate was used to label the three antibodies: anti-Stat6, anti-Phospho Rb, and an anti-GST antibody (*see* **Note 1**). The final antibody concentrations were determined using a mouse IgG as the standard. Final concentrations and labeling ratios were calculated for the three antibodies: anti-Stat6 (120 µg/mL, 5.7:1), anti-Phospho-Rb (260 µg/mL, 3.3:1), and anti-GST (530 µg/mL, 3.8:1).

1. The anti-Stat6 antibody was diluted 1:10 in PBS, and reconcentrated five times by a spin-filtration system, in order to eliminate the sodium azide (*see* **Note 1**). The other antibodies were used as received.
2. Dilute the antibodies to 1 mg/mL in carrier-protein-free and azide-free PBS.
3. Dissolve the NHS-ester ruthenium labeling reagent (M.W. 1057) in DMSO to 10 µg/mL.
4. Add to each antibody (M.W. approx 160 kDa) solution enough labeling reagent to give an 8:1 ruthenium-to-antibody molar target-labeling ratio.
5. Stir the solutions in the dark for 1 h using a small magnetic stir-bar.
6. Terminate reactions by adding 20 µL of 2 M glycine.
7. Pass the antibodies through a Sephadex G-25 column equilibrated with PBS to remove the unreacted ruthenium label.
8. Determine the ruthenium label concentration by measuring the absorbance at 455 nm ($\varepsilon = 13{,}700\ M^{-1}\text{cm}^{-1}$).
9. Determine the antibody concentration with Pierce Micro BCA kit.
10. Concentrate the antibody with a spin-filtration system as needed.

3.3. ECL Stat6/P578 Interaction Assay

The basic format of the ECL assay was kept similar to the DELFIA using the streptavidin-biotin interaction to bind the phosphopeptide to the magnetic beads, and a ruthenium labeled anti-Stat6 antibody to detect the presence of Stat6 on the beads (**Fig. 4**). Disruption of the Stat6-P578 interaction would result in less ruthenium bound to the magnetic bead and a lower ECL signal (*see* **Note 2**).

3.3.1. Assay Optimization

Preliminary experiments were carried out to establish a good signal-to-background ratio and to determine the minimum amount of the critical assay reagents required. In the initial ECL experiment, a lower amount of Stat6, higher amount of antibody, and the same amount of b-P578 were used compared with the DELFIA protocol (*see* **Note 3**). Add 25 µL of buffer, test compound, or control compound to each well (*see* **Note 4**).

1. Add 25 µL b-P578, 30 ng/well.
2. Add 25 µL of Stat6, 50 ng/well.

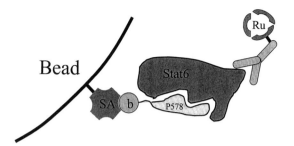

Fig. 4. Streptavidin-magnetic beads are used to capture the biotinylated phosphopeptide (b-P578). The presence of Stat6 on the bead is detected by a ruthenium labeled anti-Stat6 antibody.

3. Incubate at room temperature for 3 h.
4. Add 10 μL of ruthenium-labeled antibody, 50 ng/well.
5. Incubate at room temperature for 30 min.
6. Add 200 μL of beads, 30 μg/well.
7. Incubate at room temperature for 30 min.
8. Read with M-series Origen, or transfer well contents to tubes and read with a single-channel Origen.

To establish the initial signal window, and to check for spurious reactivity between any of the assay components, an experiment was carried out where each of the four additions was replaced by buffer. The signal measured (3.8×10^6 ECL units) from this experiment was 50 times greater than is typically necessary to obtain a good signal-to-background ratio, and negligible cross-reactivity between the assay components was observed. However, in the absence of the phosphopeptide b-P578, a signal of almost 4.9×10^5 was measured (**Fig. 5**). This signal indicates a high level of nonspecific binding of Stat6 to the beads, because a low signal (3.7×10^4) was measured in the absence of Stat6. Therefore, an initial signal window of 8:1 relative to the absence of b-P578 with a $Z' = 0.7$ was obtained. A titration of b-P578 showed a concentration dependent signal down to below 1 ng/well (**Fig. 5**).

Because of the large signals measured, the amount of the most critical reagent, Stat6, was immediately reduced fivefold to 10 ng/well, the amount used in the final protocol. Lowering the amount of Stat6 is expected to reduce the level of the background signal, because the high background is caused by nonspecific binding of Stat6 to the beads. In a further attempt to lower this nonspecific binding, a blocking agent was added to the bead suspension. A related parameter is the presence of a carrier protein (0.1% casein) in the Stat6 b-P578 buffers. The choice of carrier protein and blocking agent combination can dramatically affect the signal window of the assay. To examine this, either

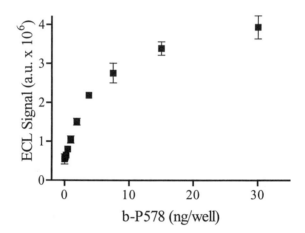

Fig. 5. Titration curve of the biotinylated P578. Each data point represents the mean of three separate measurements ± SD.

0.1% casein or 0.1% BSA was used as the carrier protein, while the blocking agents tried were casein at 0.1, 1.0, 5.0%, BSA at 0.1, 1.0, 5.0%, or undiluted Pierce Superblock. When BSA was used as the carrier protein and 5.0% casein as the blocking agent the lowest signal window (3:1) was detected. The signal window increased dramatically to 26:1 to when 0.1% casein was used as both carrier and blocking protein $Z' = 0.8$). Although Pierce Superblock gave similar results to 0.1% casein, casein is more cost-effective and was used in all buffers in subsequent experiments.

3.3.1.1. ANTIBODY TITRATION

The next most critical reagent, in terms of availability and cost after Stat6, was the ruthenium labeled anti-Stat6 antibody. To determine the optimum antibody concentration, a titration of the anti-Stat6 antibody was carried out from 50 ng/well down to 0.05 ng/well. Signal windows of 43:1, 31:1, and 15:1 were detected relative to an absence of b-P578 at 50, 12.5, and 3.1 ng/well, respectively (**Fig. 6**). A final value of 15 ng/well, reduced by a factor of two, was chosen for the ruthenium labeled anti-Stat6 antibody for all subsequent experiments.

3.3.1.2. TIME COURSE

Previously, a complicated and relatively lengthy series of incubations had been employed based on the original DELFIA assay, which required three separate incubation times totaling 4 h. However, given the nature of the assay format, one might expect that a single incubation time would be sufficient to allow the reagents to reach equilibrium in the well prior to detection. To confirm this

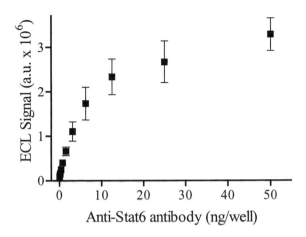

Fig. 6. Titration curve of the ruthenium-labeled anti-Stat6 antibody (*see* text for details). Each data point represents the mean of three separate measurements ± SD.

hypothesis, an experiment was performed where all four reagents were added as quickly as possible to all wells. The signal window vs an absence of b-P578 was 6:1 after 12 min, 18:1 after 60 min and 38:1 after 6 h. In previous experiments, the signal window was calculated vs an absence b-P578. For comparison, the signal window vs an excess of nonbiotinylated P578 was calculated to be 5:1 after 12 min increasing to approx 13:1 for all other times greater than 60 min. The Z' was 0.2 after 12 min, and increased to greater than 0.8 for all times greater than 60 min. The results of these experiments showed that a single incubation time with all reagents present in the well was sufficient.

3.3.1.3. BEAD TITRATION

The final experiment performed to determine the optimum reagent concentrations was a titration of the streptavidin-coated magnetic beads. At the lowest-bead concentrations, all of the beads are captured on the electrode, but some of the ruthenium-labeled reagent is not bound to the beads. Thus, a low signal would be achieved. At the intermediate concentrations, all the beads are captured on the electrode and all the ruthenium labeled reagent is bound to the beads, giving a maximum signal. Finally at the highest bead concentrations, the electrode surface becomes saturated and not all of the beads would be captured on the electrode, producing a submaximal signal. The best signal window was obtained with 30 µg/well of beads. However, the signal window was only 25% lower with 15 µg/well and a 50% saving in beads could be obtained (**Fig. 7**). Consequently, a bead concentration of 15 µg/well was used for all subsequent experiments. Even lower concentrations could possibly be used, since the Z' was greater than 0.7 for all bead concentrations, except 120 µg/well.

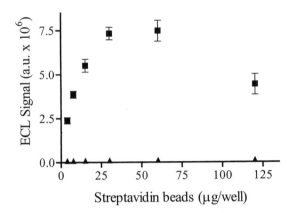

Fig. 7. Titration curve of streptavidin-coated magnetic beads. The triangles are data where b-P578 was omitted, and the squares are data with all the assay components present. Each data point represents the mean of three separate measurements ± SD.

However, using a larger signal window would help compensate for any potential increase in variability that might occur during the actual screening (*see* **Subheading 3.3.4.** for the final reagent amounts).

3.3.2. Validating the Assay

After the reagent concentrations had been established, a dose-response curve of the nonbiotinylated P578 was performed, giving values 10.9 ± 1.0 and 12.3 ± 1.0 μM in two separate experiments. These values compare well with those determined by fluorescence correlation spectroscopy (9.9 ± 1.1 μM) *(25)* and DELFIA (5.1 ± 0.8 μM) *(26)*, indicating that the assay could be expected to give acceptable results in HTS. A titration of DMSO from 0–5% of the assay volume showed no significant reduction in the signal-to-background ratio over this concentration range (*see* **Note 5**).

3.3.3 Simplifying the Final Protocol

The protocol described so far involves five sequential reagent additions: compound, b-P578, Stat6, ruthenium labeled anti-Stat6 antibody, and beads. An experiment was performed in which Stat6, b-P578, the antibody, and the beads were combined before addition to the well. This mixture was preincubated for 2 h, to allow the bead/b-P578/Stat6/Ru-antibody to interact.

1. Mix b-P578, 100 ng/mL, Stat6, 33 ng/mL, ruthenium-labeled antibody, 50 ng/mL, and beads, 50 μg/mL.
2. Incubate at room temperature for 2 h.
3. Add 10 μL of buffer, or P578 (6.3 mM) to each well.
4. Add 290 mL of mixture from **step 1**.

5. Incubate for 15 min–3 h at room temperature.
6. Transfer the contents from three wells to tubes at each time point and read with a single-channel Origen.

This experiment was performed to determine whether, once the complex had formed, the nonbiotinylated P578 could compete away the b-P578 and release the Stat6 from the bead. After 3 h, the signal had reduced to 44% of the level measured in the absence of the nonbiotinylated P578, demonstrating that P578 is unable to entirely compete away the b-P578 in this time. A second experiment was performed in which the nonbiotinylated P578 or buffer was first added to the wells, followed by Stat6, and finally a mixture of the remaining reagents, b-P578, antibody, and beads. An excellent signal-to-background of 55:1 with a Z' of 0.8 was obtained. This simplified assay was chosen as the final HTS compatible protocol for measuring the Stat6/P578 interaction with ECL.

3.3.4. VALIDATING THE FINAL PROTOCOL

Using the finalized protocol, the dose-response of the nonbiotinylated P578 was twice repeated giving 11.8 ± 1.1 μM and 11.3 ± 0.8 μM in good agreement with the previous results from the more complicated protocol, from fluorescence correlation spectroscopy (FCS), and from DELFIA (*see* above). A representative dose-response curve from the final protocol is shown in **Fig. 8**. The average of the four ECL IC_{50} determinations was 11.6 ± 1.0 μM.

1. Add 30 μL/well of test compound (10 μM final), control compound, or buffer.
2. Add 70 μL/well of Stat6,10 ng/well.
3. Add 200 μL/well of mixture of b-P578, 30 ng/well, antibody, 15 ng/well, and streptavidin-coated beads,15 ng/well.
4. Incubate 2 h at room temperature.
5. Read with M-series Origen, or transfer well contents to tubes and read with a single-channel Origen.

3.4. Additional Assay Conversion Examples

3.4.1. Myc/Max

A protein-protein interaction assay, Myc/Max, was also converted from a DELFIA assay to an ECL assay *(27)*. In order to reformat the assay for ECL, the GST or 6-His tags added to Myc and Max in order to purify the proteins were exploited to capture one protein on the magnetic beads and to label the other with ruthenium. A first attempt to format the assay employed a biotinylated anti-6-His antibody to capture the 6-His-Max onto a streptavidin-coated bead, and a ruthenium-labeled anti-GST antibody to detect the presence of GST-Myc bound to the 6-His-Max. However, control samples showed the same signal could be obtained in the absence of either 6-His-Max or GST-Myc

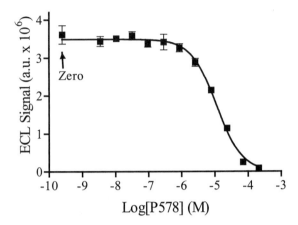

Fig. 8. A typical dose-response curve of the nonbiotinylated P578 interacting with Stat6. Each data point represents the mean of three separate measurements ± SD. Four experiments gave an average of IC_{50} of 11.6 ± 1.0 μM, when fit to a sigmoidal dose-response function with a variable slope.

as with both proteins present. Two Biacore surface-plasmon resonance experiments were used to quickly determine that there was a strong cross-reactivity between the anti-6-His antibody and the GST-Myc, and that the 6-His-Max is moderately bound to streptavidin-coated surfaces. IGEN had just completed development of a Ni-NTA coated bead, enabling the assay to be reformatted so that the 6-His-Max was captured directly by the Ni-NTA beads, and the GST-Myc bound to Max was detected with the ruthenium labeled anti-GST antibody. In this format, the assay was then optimized in very much the same way as the Stat6/P578 interaction assay giving similar results in terms of reproducible IC_{50} values, signal window, and Z' factors. These experiences suggest that care must be taken in formatting an assay with antibodies. Careful control experiments should be done very early in the assay development process to avoid wasting time working with a system that contains inherent flaws.

3.4.2. Cdk4

Tyrosine kinase assays are easily formatted for ECL with biotinylated substrates and ruthenium labeled antiphosphotyrosine antibodies like PT66 or PY20. The biotinylated substrate is bound to a streptavidin-coated magnetic bead, and the kinase activity is determined by the amount of antibody bound to the bead. The quality of such kinase assays is dependent on the quality of the antibody used. For tyrosine kinases, the antiphosphotyrosine antibodies are specific and tight binding. However, the phosphoserine and phosphothreonine epitopes for Ser/Thr kinases do not seem to offer good specific antibody recognition. For Cyclin-dependent kinase 4 (Cdk4), an Rb fragment labeled with a streptavidin recognition motif (AWRHPQFGG) was used as the substrate *(28)*, and a ruthenium-labeled antiphosphoserine-795 antibody was used to detect the kinase activity. We were able to obtain reasonable dose-response curves for several Cdk4 inhibitor compounds. However, the enzyme concentration dependent activity of the assay was linear only over a narrow range of concentrations when compared to an SPA version of the assay *(28)*. The SPA assay format did not utilize an antibody. One possible explanation for this would be that the antibody is cross-reacting with Cdk4 itself instead of recognizing the substrate. Since we did not fully understand these differences, no further optimization was done on the ECL assay. If a better antiphosphoserine antibody were available, then this format would be more likely to produce a reliable ECL assay.

4. Notes

1. If an antibody is shipped in a buffer containing a carrier protein or sodium azide, then the buffer needs to be exchanged prior to labeling to avoid reaction of the NHS ester with the carrier protein or the azide.
2. Now that Ni-NTA beads are available from IGEN, it would be possible to set up the assay to capture the His-tagged Stat6 on a Ni-NTA bead and detect the presence of the biotinylated phosphopeptide (b-P578) bound to Stat6 with ruthenium-labeled streptavidin.
3. A typical starting point for the magnetic beads is 20–30 µg/well for an ECL experiment.
4. Compounds were generally screened at 10 µ*M* final concentration, while the concentration of control compound varied depending on the potency of the control compound used.
5. DMSO is used to solubilize compounds to be tested in HTS.
6. The development of the Stat6/P578 interaction ECL assay was straightforward producing a simple-homogeneous assay feasible for HTS.
7. In comparison to the DELFIA assay, which required eleven steps including four wash steps, the ECL assay was much simpler, with only three reagent addition steps and a measurement.
8. The elimination of wash steps in the ECL assay translates to a significant reduction in the time necessary to run a full compound-library screen compared with DELFIA.
9. In general, the authors found ECL to be a sensitive nonradioactive assay method that was easy to use when developing biochemical assays for HTS.
10. A few drawbacks to ECL are that the assay volumes are large in comparison to the many methods, the read times are lengthy, and the instrumentation was often unreliable.
11. The experience gained during the evaluation of ECL allowed the authors to make a clear and informed decision about its implementation.

Acknowledgments

Charles Owens and coworkers *(23)* (Novartis) developed the original Stat6/P578-interaction assay and reagents. David Fisher (Dana Faber Institute, Boston, MA), Jennifer Lee and Dennis France *(27)* (Novartis) developed the original Myc/Max-interaction assay and reagents. Bhabatosh Chaudhauri and co-workers *(28)* (Novartis) developed the original Cdk4 assay and reagents. The authors would like to thank Linh-Chi Nguyen (Novartis) for help in editing the manuscript, and Abbie Esterman and Maura Kibbey (IGEN, Gaithersburg, MD) for their help and counseling with ECL assay development and for the first three figures.

References

1. Grimshaw, C., Gleason, C., Chojnicki, E., and Young J. (1997) Development of an equilibrium immunoassay using electrochemiluminescence detection of a novel recombinant protein product and its application to pre-clinical product development. *J. Pharm. Biomed. Res.* **16,** 605–612.
2. Jameison, F., Sanchez, R., Dong, L., Leland, J., Youst, D., and Martin M. (1996) Electrochemiluminescence-based quantitation of classical clinical chemistry analytes. *Anal. Chem.* **8,** 1298–1302.
3. Kibbey, M., Sugasawara, R., and Olson, C. (1996) Electrochemiluminescent contaminant assays: quantitation of residual protein A and BSA in bioproducts. *Biomed. Products* **21,** 136.
4. Kobrynski, L., Tanimune, L., Pawlowski, A., Douglas, S., and Campbell, D., (1996) A comparison of electrochemiluminscence and flow cytometry for the detection of natural latex-specific human Immunoglobulin E. *Clin. Diagn. Lab. Immunol.* **3,** 42–46.
5. Moreau, E., Phillipe, J., Couvent, S., and Leroux-Roels, G. (1996) Interference of soluble TNF-α receptors in immunological detection of tumor necrosis factor-α. *Clin. Chem.* **42,** 1450–1453.
6. Yu, H. and Bruno, J. (1996) Immunomagnetic-electrochemiluminescent detection of *Escherichia coli* O157 and *Salmonella typhimurium* in foods and environmental water samples. *Appl. Environ. Microbiol.* **62,** 587–592.
7. Bruno, J. G. and Yu, H. (1996) Immunomagnetic-electrochemiluminescent detection of Bacillus anthracis spores in soil matrixes. *Appl. Environ. Microbiol.* **62,** 3474–3476.
8. Gatto-Menking, D. L., Yu, H., Bruno, J. G., Goode, M. T., Miller, M., and Zulich, A. W. (1995) Sensitive detection of biotoxoids and baterial spores using an immunomagnetic electrochemiluminescence sensor. *Biosensors Bioelectron.* **10,** 501–507.
9. Christoforidis, S., Miacyzynska, M., Ashman, K., Wilm, M., Zhao, I., Yip, S., et al. (1999) Phosphatidylinositol-3-OH kinases are rab5 effectors. *Nature Cell Biol.* **1,** 249–252.

10. Liang, P., Dong, L., and Martin, M. (1996) Light emission from ruthenium-labeled penicillins signaling their hydrolysis by 3-lactamase. *J. Am. Chem. Soc.* **118,** 9198–9199.
11. Hughes, S. R., Khorkova O., Goyal, S., Knaeblein, J., Heroux, J., Riedel, N. G., and Sahasrabudhe, S. (1998) α2-macroglobulin associates with β-amyloid peptide and prevents fibril formation. *Natl. Acad. Sci.* **95,** 3275–3280.
12. Stem, H. J., Carlos, R. D., and Schutzbank, T. E. (1995) Rapid detection of the ΔF508 deletion in cystic fibrosis by allele specific PCR and electrochemiluminescence detection. *Clin. Biochem.* **28,** 470–473.
13. Kenten, J. H., Casadei, J., Link, J., Lupold, S., Willey, J., Powell, M., Rees, A., and Massey, R. (1991) Rapid electrochemiluminescence assay for polymerase chain reaction products. *Clin. Chem.* **37,** 1626–1632.
14. Bergen, A., Wang, C.-Y., Nakhai, B., and Goldman, D. (1996) Mass allele detection (MAD) of rare 5-HT1A structural variants with allele-specific amplification and electrochemiluminescent detection. *Hum. Mutat.* **7,** 135–143.
15. Schutzbank, T. E. and Smith, J. (1995) Detection of human immunodeficiency virus type I proviral DNA by PCR using an electrochemiluminescence-tagged probe. *J. Clin. Microbiol.* **33,** 2036–2041.
16. Abraham, R., Buxbaum, S., Link, J., Smith, R., Venti, C., and Darsley, M. (1996) Determination of binding constants of diabodies directed against prostate-specific antigen using electrochemiluminescence-based immunoassays. *J. Mol. Recog.* **9,** 456–461.
17. Koumanov, F., Yang, J., Jones, A., Hatanaka, Y., and Homan, G. (1998) Cell-surface biotinylation of GLUT4 using bis-mannose photolabels. *Biochem. J.* **330,** 1209–1215.
18. Fantuzzi, G., Sacco, S., Ghezzi, P., and Dinarello, C. (1997) Physiological and cytokine responses in IL-1β-deficient mice after zymosan-induced inflammation. *Am. J. Physiol.* **273,** R400–R406.
19. Zacchi, P., Stenmark, H., Parton, R., Orioli, D., Lim, F., Giner, A., et al. (1998) Rab17 regulates membrane trafficking through apical recycling endosomes in polarized epthelial cells. *J. Cell Biol.* **140,** 1039–1053.
20. Simonsen, A., Lippe, R., Christoforidis, S., Gaullier, J., Brech, A., Gallaghan, J., et al. (1998) EEA1 links PI(3)K function to Rab5 regulation of endosome fusion. *Nature* **394,** 494–498.
21. Yang, H., Leland, J. K., Yost, D., and Massey, R. J. (1994) Electrochemiluminescence: A new diagnostic and research tool. *Bio/Technol.* **12,** 193–194.
22. Deaver, D. R. (1995) A new non-isotopic detection system for immunoassays. *Nature* **377,** 758–760.
23. Graham, B., Head, D., Jones, C., and Owen, C. (1997) Expression, purification and characterisation of latent Stat6. *Novartis Internal Report*, PKF-97-03588.
24. Zhang, J.-H., Chung, T. D. Y., and Oldenburg, K. R. (1999) A simple statistical parameter for use in evaluation and validation of high throughput screening assays. *J. Biomol. Screen.* **4,** 67–73.

25. Mueller, K., Schilb, A., Auer, M., Jones, C., Owen, C., and Stoeckli, K. (1999) The interaction of Stat6 with phospho-tyrosine peptides: a homogeneous solution assay based on fluorescence correlation spectroscopy. *Novartis Internal Report*, PKF-99-00270.
26. Chin M. Personal communication.
27. Lee, J., Kennon, S.-C., Clune, K., and France, D. (1999) Development of a high-throughput screening assay to discover antagonists of Myc/Max interaction. *Novartis Internal Report*, RD-2000-50429.
28. Wu, J., Yarwood, D. R., Chaudhuri, B., Muller, L., Zurini, M., and Sills, M. A. (2000) Measurement of Cdk4 kinase activity using an affinity peptide-tagging technology. *Comb. Chem. High Throughput Screen* **3,** 27–36.

6

Cellular Assays in HTS

Patricia Johnston

1. Introduction

Cell-based screens represent one of the most venerable approaches to lead generation, indeed, antimicrobial screens were the mainstay of drug discovery in the 1940s, 1950s, and 1960s *(1)*. However, cellular assays also represent one of the most dynamic areas of innovation in high-throughput screening (HTS). The driver of this innovation is the demand for more leads from more complex targets. Genomics discovery efforts have generated many potential targets for HTS, but the biochemical nature of these novel targets may not be elucidated prior to their entry into the lead generation process. Therefore, these targets are frequently addressed in "gene to screen" paradigms that rely on cellular-screening approaches. Advances in cell-based screening approaches have also been driven by the need to address complex, multi-component target classes that may not be feasible in biochemical assays. Finally, the increasingly combative intellectual property playing field, and the need to accelerate the drug discovery process have driven innovations in cell-based screening methodologies.

The purpose of this chapter is to review cell-based screening methodologies currently in widespread use in the HTS laboratory. For the sake of brevity, I will focus only on eukaryotic systems, although there have been many recent advances in the screening of microbial systems both for the purposes of target validation *(2)* and lead generation *(3,4)* . Likewise, I will only discuss those methods that are compatible with HTS, in other words, cellular assays that support a minimal daily throughput of 5,000 samples.

From: *Methods in Molecular Biology, vol. 190: High Throughput Screening: Methods and Protocols*
Edited by: W. P. Janzen © Humana Press Inc., Totowa, NJ

2. Why Bother?

Cellular assay systems can be more complex and less well-defined than biochemical assays, and in some instances are more expensive and labor-intensive as well. So, why bother configuring a cell-based assay for HTS? The answers lie in the drug discovery strategy deployed for that target class and in the nature of the biological target. Drug discovery strategies focused on novel, potentially orphan targets require that screens be configured for targets for which the mechanism of action and relevance to disease have not been elucidated. In many such cases, the results of the HTS are expected to drive the validation of the target. Arguably, for these poorly characterized targets, a screen in which the target is expressed and regulated in a cellular environment ensures that the necessary substrates and cofactors of that target are available at physiologically appropriate concentrations. Thus, cellular assays negate the need to determine the appropriate cofactors, etc., prior to HTS. However, a cell-based approach may also be desirable for well-defined targets with clear disease relevance. For example, in cases where the molecular target is difficult or expensive to express and purify at the scale needed for HTS, a cell-based assay may represent the fastest, least expensive approach.

Complex targets which are very challenging to reconstitute in a biochemical assay represent another opportunity for cellular HTS applications. These would include targets that regulate a signaling pathway, e.g., the SOCS proteins, targets that are themselves regulated by poorly understood partners in a signaling pathway, or targets that require assembly of a regulatory complex. These targets are best screened in a cellular system in which all of the necessary components are pre-assembled.

In addition, cell-based screens may provide the means to identify compounds with a unique mechanism of action, for example, agonist or allosteric modulator of G-protein-coupled receptor (GPCR) targets. Finally, cellular HTS approaches may circumvent intellectual property restrictions on use of the cDNA for a target if a cell line is available that already expresses the gene of interest.

To summarize, though cell-based HTS may initially appear daunting, there are many targets for which a cell-based screen represents the fastest, cheapest path to lead generation. Furthermore, the complexity of cell-based assays may enable discovery of compounds with unique mechanisms of action. Certainly, cell-based screens ensure that intracellular targets are expressed in the appropriate physiological context and that active compounds have a favorable permeability profile.

3. Potential Cellular "Platforms"

The cellular platform or background chosen to approach a particular target has an enormous impact both on the development and the implementation of a HTS for that target. The choices are extensive, and include primary cell types and cell lines; both "native" and engineered. The choice is driven by the availability and behavior of the cells, as well as the amplitude and reproducibility of the signal attainable in that cellular system. Primary cells of human origin are the most physiologically relevant lead generation platform. Selected primary human cell types are commercially available and amenable to HTS *(5)* (Clonetics, Walkersville, MD), and various rodent primary cell types can be prepared at HTS scale. However, in general, primary cells cannot be obtained at the scale necessary for HTS. Thus, primary cell screens are typically positioned in the screening paradigm as low-throughput secondary assays.

Transformed cell lines of human origin are the most commonly used cell-based screening platform. These lines can be screened in their "native" state for targets naturally expressed in these cells, e.g., neuropeptide receptors expressed in the SK-N-MC neuroblastoma line *(6)*. Many of these lines retain a highly differentiated phenotype and are an excellent platform on which to screen a complex physiological response, such as secretion, e.g., insulin secretion from insulinoma lines *(7)*. Certain native cell lines serve as platforms in which to study the differentiation process itself. In these screens, a cocktail of stimuli is used to drive the cells down a differentiation path; an aspect of this differentiation process can be screened, or the terminally differentiated cells can be used to screen a particular physiological process. There are many cell lines amenable to differentiation studies; commonly used lines include C_2C_{12} *(8)*, U937 *(9)*, and L6 *(10)* cells.

Cell lines can be further engineered to express or over-express a target of interest. Some assay formats require co-expression of multiple proteins, or expression of "reporter" proteins. Expression can be transient or stable, and a number of expression systems employed, depending on the nature of the cell line and the target. Stable cell lines are most commonly generated by plamid transfection or retroviral infection. Plasmids can be introduced to the cell by internalization of DNA precipitates, electroporation, or DNA-liposome fusion (lipofection). Electroporation is the method of choice for suspension cultures, while lipofection is commonly employed for adherent cells. Clones can be isolated, or pooled cell populations can be utilized for HTS. Retroviral systems, in which the target DNA is introduced by viral infection are an attractive alternative to plasmid transfection, obviate the clonal selection step and can generate lines with high target expression levels.

Stable expression of the target is perhaps the easiest choice for HTS, but transient expression can be scaled up sufficiently to support a reasonable throughput. Transient transfection procedures generate a population of cells with generally high levels of target expression. Should isolation of a stable clone prove difficult, transient expression of a target may represent the fastest path to HTS. Batch lipofection is easily scaled-up and highly reproducible, but the reagents can be expensive for a full HTS campaign.

4. Common Cell-Based HTS Formats

Perhaps one of the oldest and most widely used eukaryotic HTS formats is the reporter assay *(7)*. Reporter assays can be designed to detect the transcriptional regulation of a particular gene, or they can be configured to detect activity of a signaling pathway. In reporter assays, the expression of a protein whose enzymatic activity is easily detected is linked to the biological activity of the target of interest. Transcriptional regulation reporter assays are configured by linking the promoter, or elements of the promoter, from the gene of interest to the coding region of the reporter gene. To detect activity of a signaling pathway, repeats of a particular response element are queued upstream of the reporter gene and regulate its expression in response to activation of the pathway. Potential reporter proteins include; chloramphenical acetyl transferase, firefly and renilla luciferase, secreted human growth hormone, β-galactosidase, secreted alkaline phosphatase, green fluorescent protein(s), (GFPs), and β-lactamase *(12)*. Of these, luciferase, β-galactosidase, and β-lactamase reporters are the most commonly used in HTS laboratories.

There are both advantages and disadvantages to reporter screens. Widespread implementation of this assay format has driven the development of multiple instrumentation platforms and a diversity of reagent kits compatible with them. The cost of reagents for reporter screens, though not low, is acceptable, and many of the commercially available reagents provide advantages such as greater signal amplitude or stability. Most importantly, reporter screens are highly amenable to miniaturization *(13)*.

Reporter screens have their limitations as well. Reporter gene transcription triggered by receptor activation generates an indirect signal removed both spatially and temporally from the target. One could argue that this indirect and amplified signal might obscure subtle modulation of the receptor. For example, reporters designed to detect Gs-coupled receptor activity are often configured to amplify the signal via multiple copies of the cAMP response element. Such amplification can result in unusual dose-dependent pharmacology *(14)*. Reporter assays designed to detect the activity of receptors that signal via calcium mobilization typically utilize the NFAT-response element. However,

NFAT-mediated gene expression is dependent on both the amplitude and duration of the calcium flux *(15)*, and therefore NFAT-driven reporter assays cannot be used to detect rapid calcium-mediated responses. For these reasons it may be desirable to design screens that detect signaling events more proximal to the receptor, such as receptor phosphorylation, G-protein recruitment, cAMP generation, or calcium mobilization.

HTS of cellular calcium mobilization was greatly facilitated by the introduction of the FLIPR (Molecular Devices, Sunnyvale, CA), a fluorescent-imaging system that collects information about the calcium flux in each well of a microplate (both 96- and 384-well) simultaneously *(16)*. Intracellular calcium concentrations are measured by preloading the cells with a calcium-sensitive fluorescent dye, such as Fluo3 *(17)*. FLIPR reads at subsecond intervals, which enables capture of the response kinetics. This feature, along with the liquid-handling capabilities of the device, facilitates identification of subtle effects on receptor activity, and successive liquid additions enable discrimination of agonist, allosteric modulation, and antagonist activity within the same plate of cells.

Obviously, cell-based screens designed to detect calcium mobilization are limited to those receptors that signal through this pathway. Co-expression of a promiscuous (Gα15, Gα16), or chimeric G protein can "switch" the signal of GPCRs so that they couple to InsP$_3$ generation and calcium release *(18)*. These G-protein switching strategies have made calcium-mobilization screening approaches applicable to many more receptors. However, screens designed to detect receptor activity against a backdrop of stable, high-level promiscuous G protein expression are often susceptible to artifacts: false-positives derived presumably from other cell-surface receptors hi-jacking the G protein.

Although the FLIPR has facilitated advances in calcium-mobilization screens, these assays remain difficult to configure, relatively slow, and fraught with potential artifacts. The optics of the device limit fluorescence detection to the bottom of the well. This reduces background fluorescence, but also requires that the cells be firmly adhered. If the cells detach or move during liquid addition, the signal is compromised. Likewise, the best signal is obtained from densely seeded wells, which can generate large cell-culture requirements for implementation in the high-throughput laboratory.

Other signaling events proximal to the receptor can be screened including: receptor phosphorylation, dimerization, or internalization; cAMP-generation; or G protein recruitment. Of these approaches, cAMP-detection assays are the most amenable to HTS. These screens are designed to detect cAMP levels present in the cell 30–60 min after receptor activation. The cells are lysed and the cAMP level quantified, typically by an immuno-assay. Numerous kits are marketed for cAMP quantitation on multiple-assay platforms, including radioactive (Amersham Pharmacia Biotech, Uppsala Sweden, or NEN Life Sciences Inc, Boston MA), luminescent (Tropix, or Biosignal, Montreal Canada), and fluorescent-assay systems (LJL Biosystems, Sunnyvale CA). The advantages of cAMP generation screens are related to the assay format and the nature of the target. Some of these assay systems are homogenous and amenable to miniaturization, others are compatible only with 96-well plates. All of the assays are fairly expensive. The most significant disadvantage of this approach is apparent in screens of receptors linked to Gi. These screens are frequently limited by a small dynamic range of signal.

Reporter, cAMP, or calcium-mobilization screens are ideally suited for the identification of agonist activities, but antagonist identification does not require a cellular assay. Typically, antagonist screens are configured as binding assays utilizing isolated receptors or membrane preparations. However, cell-based approaches to antagonist identification can be attractive alternatives to biochemical binding assays. Cell-based ligand-binding assays can be configured with scintillant-impregnated plates (Cytostar T plates, Amersham Life Sciences, Arlington Heights, IL; Flashplates, NEN Life Science Products Inc, Boston, MA). Cellular monolayers are established in the wells and radiolabeled ligand is added to the media. Binding to the surface receptor excites the scintillant via a proximity effect, and the radiolabel in solution is silent. This approach removes the need to prepare membranes, thereby reducing the cell-culture requirements for HTS, and reduces the number of wash steps required with membrane-binding assays. Furthermore, the short compound-incubation periods obviate the cytotoxicity complications present in other assay formats such as reporter screens designed to detect antagonist activity.

Cell-based proximity assays have also proven useful to screening transporters. Cell-based screens for transporter targets, such as amino acid or neurotransmitter carriers, are preferred when ligand binding to the transporter is complicated by either high nonspecific binding by sticky ligands, or low expression of the transporter. Additionally, cell-based approaches to transporter targets enable identification of allosteric modulators that might be missed in a binding assay.

Proliferation assays are another common cell-based screening format in which scintillant-impregnated plates can be used. Proliferation assays can be configured to address a wide diversity of targets that either stimulate or inhibit cell growth: including cell-surface growth factor or cytokine receptors, intracellular enzymes, or multidrug-resistance pumps. Direct quantitation of ^{14}C-thymidine incorporation into DNA provides one of the most sensitive assays for cellular proliferation. Likewise, assays designed to quantify protein synthesis by detection of ^{35}S-methioine incorporation are one of the most sensitive methods to detect cytotoxic compounds. The scintillant-impregnated plates described above enable both of these assays. However, the radioactive nature of these screens can make them a less attractive choice for HTS than fluorescent or colorimetric approaches utilizing tetrazolium dyes such as WST1, MTT, or XTT (Boehringer Mannheim Biochemicals).

Finally, cell-based assays can be designed to measure changes in protein expression. These screens can be configured to quantify protein expression on the cell surface, within the cell, or secreted into the medium via immunocytochemical techniques *(5,19)*. The signal is determined by the modification of the secondary antibodies; fluorescent and colorimetric formats are available and compatible with multiple instrumentation platforms. Implementation of these approaches is of course dependent on the availability of an antibody specific for the protein(s) of interest. These screens are straightforward to develop and typically inexpensive, but are hindered by the need for multiple wash steps. Changes in protein expression can also be monitored by detection of mRNA expression. However, assays to quantify changes in mRNA expression have not been implemented at a high-throughput scale *(20,21)*.

5. Implementation Challenges

Cell-based screens generate unique challenges for HTS implementation. These challenges arise during the development and validation of cell-based screens and continue through implementation in HTS during which the cell culture must be scaled to support daily production of hundreds of microplates for a campaign of weeks or months duration. Implementation challenges tied to the nature of cell culture at scale are beyond the scope of this review. Key challenges tied to cell-based screen development, regardless of the assay format, include the growth and adherence properties of the cells, solvent tolerance, cytotoxicity complications, and the stability of the cellular phenotype.

Growth and adherence issues are at the heart of many assay reproducibility problems. In screens dependent on long incubation periods (24–48 h), variations in cell growth across the plate can generate significant signal drift that usually manifests as edge effects. This differential growth is typically due to temperature variations or media evaporation, and can be controlled by careful regulation of the humidity and temperature of the incubator chambers, and by ensuring that the microplates are distributed evenly in the incubators. Poor or inconsistent cellular adherence can also produce significant variation in the signal of certain assay formats. Screen formats particularly prone to cellular adherence artifacts include calcium mobilization assays utilizing FLIPR, cellular enzyme-linked immunosorbent assays (ELISAs), or other assays in which the cell monolayers must be washed, and any assay requiring removal and transfer of incubation media. Poor adherence can be improved by coating the surface of the microplate with a charged substrate such as poly-lysine or with extracellular matrix components such as fibronectin or collagen. Coated plates are commercially available, or plates can be prepared in-house at reasonable expense.

Solvent and compound intolerances as evidenced by cytotoxicity are more difficult challenges to address. In general, solvents such as dimethyl sulfoxide (DMSO) interfere with cell-based assays at concentrations of 1% or less. Higher seeding densities or serum concentration can mitigate these effects slightly, but a low solvent tolerance may be inherent to a cellular platform. Likewise, cytotoxicity complications apparent in assays that require long incubation periods are inevitable, and in many cases can only be addressed by changing the assay configuration or by a secondary assay triage protocol.

6. Future of Cell-Based Screening

The two drivers of innovation in cell-based screening methodologies are the need to miniaturize and the desire to capture temporal and spatial data on target activity: "high-content" screens. Miniaturization refers both to efforts focused on scaling to smaller well volumes; 96, 384, 1536, etc., but also to different screening platforms such as microfluidics that minimize reagent needs. The challenges associated with smaller well volumes are amplified versions of those apparent with any microplate-based cell assay, i.e., cell growth, adherence, solvent tolerance, etc. One unique challenge to lower volume screening is cell seeding, particularly for adherent cells. Smaller well volumes can increase bubbling or impede even liquid distribution across the bottom of the well, both of which can result in uneven cell attachment. This challenge is tied directly to the state of the art in liquid handling instrumentation, and will evolve as these instruments evolve. Cell-based screening on chips, however, is rich with unique implementation challenges and opportunities. Chip technologies such as those available from Caliper Technologies (Caliper Technologies Corp., Mt. View CA), require fewer cells and have the potential for rapid ligand challenge and read times. These properties generate opportunities for screening of primary cells and may enable screening of transient events such as channel activity.

High content screening, such as that enabled by Cellomics technology (Pittsburg PA), though not compatible with high throughput, represents a trend in cell-based screening towards capture of richer data on more complex aspects of target activity *(22)*. These technologies enable direct visualization, in real-time if desired, of target movement in the cell, and represent unique methods to study receptor activity or transcriptional regulation.

7. Conclusion

Cell-based high throughput screens are a powerful tool in the lead generation process. Cellular assays though potentially challenging can represent the fastest path to lead identification for novel, poorly characterized targets. A cellular approach provides insight into the permeability profile of the active compounds and enables identification of compounds with unique mechanisms of action. Recent advances in the instrumentation applicable to cellular screening have enabled closer examination of the intricacies of intracellular signaling events. These advances suggest that cellular approaches will prove as fruitful a source of new leads in the twenty-first century as the antimicrobial screens were for the last.

References

1. Drews, J. (2000) Drug discovery: a historical perspective. *Science* **287,** 1960–1964.
2. Martin, M. J., Dekisi, J. L., Bennett, H. M. (1998) Drug target validation and identification of secondary drug targets using microarrays. *Nature Med.* **4,** 1293–1301.
3. Klein, R. D. and Geary, T. G. (1997) Recombinant microorganism as tools for high throughput screening for nonantibiotic compounds. *J. Biomol. Screening* **2,** 41–49.
4. Beydon, M., Fournier, A., Drugenult, L., et al. (2000) Microbiological high throughput screening, an opportunity for the lead discovery process. *J. Biomol. Screening* **5,** 13–21.
5. Rice, J. W., Davis, J. E., Crowl, R. M., et al. (1996) Development of a high volume screen to identify inhibitors of endothelial cell activation. *Anal. Biochem.* **241,** 254–259.
6. Drake, Ajayi, A., Lowe, S. R., et al., (1998) Desensitization of CGRP and adrenomedullin receptors in SK-N-MC cells: implications for the RAMP hypothesis. *Endocrinology* **140,** 533–537.
7. Clarke, S. A., Quande, C., Constandy, H., et al. (1997) Novel insulinoma cell lines produced by iterative engineering of glut2, glukokinase, and human insulin expression. *Diabetes* **46,** 958–967.
8. Yaffe, D. and Saxel, O. (1977) Serial passaging and differentiation of myogenic cells isolated from dystrophic mouse muscle. *Nature* **270,** 725–727.
9. Koren, H. S., Anderson, S. J., and Larrick, J. W. (1979) In vitro activation of a human macrophage-like cell line. *Nature* **279,** 328–331.
10. Yaffe, D. (1968) Retention of differentiation potentialities during prolonged cultivation of myogenic cells. *PNAS* **61,** 477–483.
11. Dhundale, A. and Goddard, C. (1996) Reporter assays in the high throughput screening laboratory; a rapid and robust first look. *J. Biomol. Screening* **1,** 115–118.

12. Zlokarnik, G., Negulescu, P. A., Knapp, T. E., et al. (1998) Quantitation of transcription and clonal selection of single living cells with beta-lactamase reporter. *Science* **279,** 84–88.
13. Comley, J., Reeves, T., and Robinson, P. (1998) A 1536 colorimetric SEAP reporter assay: comparison with 96- and 384 well formats. *J. Biomol. Screening* **3,** 217–226.
14. George, S., Bungay, P., and Naylor, L. (1997) Evaluation of a CRE-directed luciferase reporter gene assay as an alternative to measuring cAMP accumulation. *J. Biomol. Screening* **4,** 235–240.
15. Dolmetsch, R. E., Lewis, R. S., Goodnow, C. C., et al. (1997) Differential activation of transcription factors induced by Ca^{+2} response amplitude and duration. *Nature* **386,** 855–858.
16. Schroeder, K. and Neagle, B. S. (1996) FLIPR: a new instrument for accurate, high throughput optical screening. *J. Biomol. Screening* **1,** 75–80.
17. Minta, A., Kao, J. P., and Tsien, R. Y. (1989) Fluorescent indicators for cytosolic calcium based on rhodamine and fluorescein chromophores. *J. Biol. Chem.* **264,** 8171–8178.
18. Offermans, S. and Simon, M. I. (1995) G alpha 15 and G alpha 16 couple a wide variety of receptors to phospholipase C. *J. Biol. Chem.* **270,** 15,175–15,180.
19. DeWit et al. (1998) Large scale screening assay for the phosphorylation of mitogen-activated protein kinase in cells. *J. Biomol. Screening* **3,** 277–284.
20. Surry, D., McAllister, G., Meneses-Lorente, G., et al. (1999) High throughput ribonuclease protection assay for the determination of CYP3A mRNA induction in cultured rat hepatocytes. *Xenobiotica* **8,** 827–838.
21. Hahn, S. E., Yu, M., Tong, S., et al. (1999) Development of an in vitro screening assay for compounds that increase bone formation. *J. Biomol. Screening* **4,** 363–371.
22. Conway, Minor, L. K., Xu, J. Z., et al. (1999) Quantification of G-protein coupled receptor internalization using G-protein coupled receptor-green fluorescent protein conjugates with the ArrayScan high-content screening system. *J. Biomol. Screening* **4,** 75–86.

7

Compound Library Management

James A. Chan and Juan A. Hueso-Rodríguez

1. Introduction

The growing number of compounds synthesized and screened in the pharmaceutical industry due to the rapid development of high-throughput chemistry and screening technologies are a response to the need of more and better quality compounds in the industry pipelines. But these inmense collections (from several hundred thousands to several millions of compounds) pose a tremendous logistical problem to be overcome in order to harvest all their tremendous potential. Some reviews have appeared to deal with this topic (*1,2*), but an update seemed necessary due to the rapid evolution of this field. The scope of this chapter is the management of different types of compound collections from both physical and electronic points of view, including some aspects of natural product-extracts collections. This management is a very difficult and demanding process involving the use of sophisticated equipment and databases. The first thing to bear in mind when implementing this process is that a specialized and dedicated group should be created to be responsible for maintaining the collection and processing the orders or requests from the rest of the company. Failure to do so usually ends up with a chaotic situation where no samples can be retrieved in due time and proper format, with no control on the available amounts and locations of the samples. Proper management of the compound collection is the foundation of a quality screening organization. If this function does not operate properly, the most advanced assay technologies will fail to afford reproducible lead compounds.

From: *Methods in Molecular Biology, vol. 190: High Throughput Screening: Methods and Protocols*
Edited by: *W. P. Janzen* © Humana Press Inc., Totowa, NJ

2. Types of Collections and Stores

The sources of compounds used in a screening program are the company's historical collection, new chemical entities prepared for the current projects, prospective or unbiased chemical libraries prepared by combinatorial or parallel synthesis and, finally, external purchases.

The compounds in a collection can be stored in two different ways: neats (usually as solids) and solutions. The most common situation in any high-throughput screening (HTS) group is to both store solids and solutions if sufficient compound is available. The obvious reason is that solutions in plates are more suited for HTS even though neats are more stable under long-term storage conditions. Solids in pre-tared bar-coded vials are normally stored at room temperature, usually in automated stores. They should be easily retrievable for confirmation of activity, secondary testing, and structural verification. Compounds in solution are stored in plates or tubes, typically at two different concentrations. One is a high concentration solution (10–5 mM) in vials or plates at low temperature (4° to –20°C) for preparing lower concentration plates for HTS, long-range storage, and used as a repository and/or for dose-response experiments. The other one is a lower concentration solution in plates (1–0.1 mM) at temperatures ranging from ambient to –20°C used as a source for primary and secondary screening. In some cases, two sets of the lower concentration plates are prepared, one kept at low temperature for long-range storage, and a second one as a working set at ambient or slightly below temperatures. This second collection usually is date stamped and a shelf life is assigned after which the set is discarded and substituted for a new one.

When the collection is from natural-products extracts, all that was described previously can be applied, just substituting neat compounds by dried extracts and the compound solutions by extract solutions. In this case, absolute concentration cannot be determined since we do not know the components of the extract and their quantities present, but a relative concentration can be used just by taking original concentrations in the fermentation broth as the unit. In case of plants, marine organisms, or other materials, the initial concentration usually is in the range of 10–1 mg/mL of dried extract.

The stores used for all these types of collections can vary from shelves in a cold room to independent freezers or containers that are kept at the designed temperature. In some cases, humidity conditions are also controlled and even inert atmospheres are used. All these require manual input and output of the samples which is resource extensive and very prone to mistakes. To solve this problem, large automated stores have been devised and are now available in the market. These systems are described in the following chapter. Nevertheless, for small and medium size collections as those generated *de novo* for

starting an HTS program or the historic collections of small pharma companies, intermediate solutions can be applied that combine an automated storage
system with the basic liquid-handling required for all these systems.

Liquid handling is a critical component of any storage system and should be
capable of producing the samples in the formats required by the HTS systems,
like plate density (96-, 384-, or 1536-well plates), controls and standards positions, amounts, concentrations, single- or multiple-well replicates and dose-
response formats. This require to have systems capable of dispensing liquids
from few nanoliters to several microliters with high accuracy, precision, and
adequate throughput so they are able to provide the samples in a timely manner. The usual requirements are at least one system for dissolving dry compounds from vials to the appropriate concentration, another system for plate
replication and reformatting, and a third system with the ability to cherry pick
rows, individual wells or tubes to create adhoc plates for mixture deconvolution
or dose-response analysis. The number of these systems can then be scaled-up
or combined into one single platform commensurate with the collection size
and the throughput required by the HTS process. Examples of the equipment
available in the market for all the tasks described in this and remaining sections
can be found in the Appendix at the end of the chapter.

2.1. Processing of Compounds

As an example of the processing of compounds for different types of orders,
we present here the procedure followed at GlaxoSmithKline and graphically
schematized in **Fig. 1**. Samples are processed for therapeutic teams and HTS
based on whether compounds are prepared by traditional synthetic methods or
parallel synthesis. Compounds prepared by traditional methods are registered,
submitted in pre-tared barcoded vials, entered into inventory and 1–2 mg solid
weighed out immediately and submitted to the therapeutic team for testing.
Another sample enough to make 1–2 mL of 10 mM DMSO solution will also
be weighed out into a vial, dissolved, and dispensed into a plate. Compounds
prepared by parallel synthesis use an in-house database that track the design,
synthesis, purification, quality control (QC), registration, and submission into
inventory in a per library basis. The molecular weight and weight can then be
downloaded as text file into a liquid handler with spanable tips, e.g., Tecan
Genesis or CCS/Packard Multiprobe and appropriate amount of dimethyl sulfoxide (DMSO) added to the vials to make 10 mM solution. Aliquots can then
be transferred into a stock plate for the preparation of 1 mM source plates.
These source plates are then used to dispense compounds into different types
of screening plates based on the different assay requirements. There are
numerous liquid handlers in the market with 96 or 384 heads that can dispense

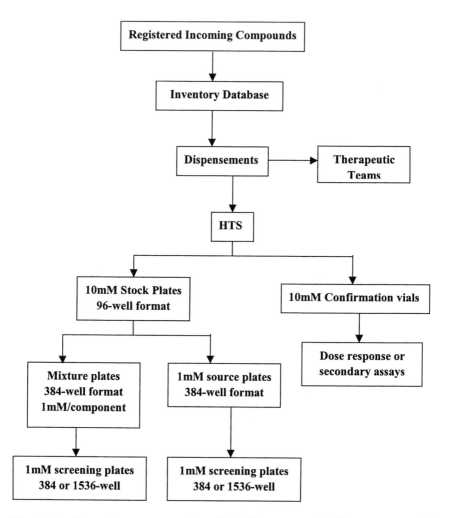

Fig. 1. A schematic representation of the Process on the Management of the Compound Collection is shown.

volumes as low as 50 nL into 384- or 1536-well plates for HTS, e.g., Robbins Hydra/Tango and CCS/Packard PlateTrack. The remaining volume in the vials is reserved for dose-response analysis and structural verification. The vials and plates can then be stored in stand-alone freezers and processed using stand-alone liquid handlers with stackers or stored in automatic refrigerated stores like Tecan's Molbank that carries its own integrated liquid-handler dispensing unit. For very large collections there are now automated liquid stores in the market that store plates and vials integrated with all types of liquid handlers needed to process plates for HTS and cherry pick vials for dose-response analysis in very high throughputs.

3. Informatic Tools

As it can be clearly seen from the previous section, the management of such huge collections with a tremendous variety of demands can not be done without the help of an Inventory Database, not only to being able to process all the types of incoming orders and outgoing samples and plates but also to keep track of all the samples locations, current amounts, and dispensement history for solids or solutions. The Inventory Database should be linked to other informations of much interest such as lot identification, source, reference to the obtaintion procedure, molecular weight, molecular formula, structure, program, or project the compound was originally prepared for, submission date, inventory entry date and internal identification number and QC data. In the specific case of natural-products extracts other information like producing organism (taxonomy), part or tissue used for the extraction, method of extraction, geographical origin of the organism, method of cultivation, etc., should be added. It is important to note that the more information kept for any given sample, the better, but trying not to overload the database so its use and maintenance is kept at a reasonable level. Another important issue is the interface of this Database, whose use for data entry should be restricted to a limited number of people due to its complexity and the high value of the information stored. This is usually solved through an intermediate interface where scientists can enter their orders to be then processed by Compound Bank staff.

3.1. Requesting of Compounds

A Lotus Notes Database is used by the Therapeutic Teams to request compounds in solid or solution form for testing. This database is critical in tracking the status of the compound request especially for a large organization with different research sites in different countries. This database has automatic notification feature via e-mail for both the requester and recipient when the request is completed. The requester can check for availability of compounds in solution or solid form using another in-house database accessible through desktop PCs that also allows the scientist to query published biological and physical data. This request database also tracks the compounds from the time they leave the Compound Bank to the time they reach the recipient's laboratory. For a list of compounds, a dispensement barcode will be provided and the recipient can scan the barcode to generate a spreadsheet enumerating pertinent information (e.g., compound number, molecular weight, amount dispensed, barcode, etc.) in order to prepare the testing solutions. This database has the following required fields for the requester:

Requested by: Name of the requestor.

Requested for: Name of the recipient if different to the requestor.

Department: Name of department.

Ship to site: Specific location where the samples should be shipped.

Program/Project name: Program name or code.

List of compounds: Internal numbers of the compounds requested (Chemical names are not admitted, since the Inventory Database only recognize the internal codes.)

Quantity needed: Amount required. (Normally 1–2 mg for solids or 20 μL of a 10 mM DMSO solution. Requester has to justify request when amount exceeds the norm.)

DMSO solution acceptable? Only for those cases where not solid is available.

Compounds checked against Inventory: Availabilities checked prior to sending the order (This process is highly recommended in order to avoid the iterative cycles of questioning if solutions and amounts are acceptable, delaying the processing of the order.)

Purpose: General and short description on what the samples are intended for (for tracking purposes only.)

Attach a file: For Excel or text attachments.

Comments: General comments on urgency or specific requirements. The Compound Bank personnel is required to complete the following fields:

Responsible person: Name of the person that processes the order.

Dispatch date: For requests outside the site. The requester and recipient are automatically notified via e-mail when a dispatch date is typed in.

Shipment number: Needed to track the shipment.

Ready for pickup: For requests within the same site. The requester and recipient are automatically notified via e-mail when the samples are ready for pickup.

The complexity of this Database varies directly with the complexity of the research organization due to the number and types of requests.

3.2. Tracking of Compounds in Plates and Vials

The Inventory Database is central to the purpose of tracking compounds on a vial/plate/well basis by assigning a barcode to each container, e.g., the stock plate is a container and has a barcode and every well/compound in this particular plate is also assigned a barcode. It is important to track the compound into the well basis, as the integrity of each sample might be different due to different storage condition and usage. The inventory database is linked to the registration database that contains all the relevant compound properties and the screening database, which contains all the biological results. The main customer of the Compound Bank is usually the Screening Departments. For primary screening, scientists generate a request indicating which plates are required to carry out a specific screening run. These plates are barcoded and then provided to the Compound Bank for assay-plate dispensement. The source plates used for the dispensation are in 384-well format containing 50 µL of a 1 mM solution in neat DMSO. These plates exist in the inventory database and volumes are debited on dispensement. The volume normally requested ranges from 300 nL to 1 µL, and thus these source plates have enough volume for 30–40 screens. Dose-response analysis and structural-verification samples are retrieved from vials containing a 10 mM solution in neat DMSO and the volume normally requested ranges from 5–10 µL and dispensed directly into the first column (for 96-well plates) or the first two columns (for 384-well plates) of plates suitable for serial dilution and IC_{50}s determination or for liquid chromatography/mass spectometry (LC/MS) structural integrity analysis. A barcode is generated for each sample using the inventory database and these barcodes are imported to the screening or analytical database as sample IDs. The barcode system allows the screening or analytical team to quickly access data necessary to assay the plate and calculate raw data to generate results. The available volume for the 10 mM source (vial or plate) is debited upon dispensements.

4. QC of the Collection

A very important issue, usually overlooked when starting a compound collection, is the quality of the compounds introduced into it. It is very important that the compounds that enter the collection are checked to verify that they comply with a certain requirement of purity and integrity. Only misleading results can be expected for a collection with compounds with very different or poor levels of purity. The second issue is that many compounds slowly degrade and that the stability is highly dependent on the storage conditions, but at the same time there is no existing storage method that can guarantee no decomposition of the compounds in the collection. It is clear then that any hit from the HTS should be considered as preliminary until a confirmation of the integrity of the screening sample has been obtained.

4.1. QC of Screening Hits

One of the key steps after the finding of active compounds with desirable chemical and biological properties is the structural verification of these hits. The source of these samples for QC could either be a sample of the solution from the confirmation vial or a sample of the solid if available, or both. It is important to track the sample to container level with dispensement barcode. Ideally, when screening hits are reported to the team, the information submitted should include not only activity but also recently obtained physical QC data. With the advent of parallel synthesis, solids normally are not available for confirmation of activity and structure and in these cases, solution samples are used. If even this type of samples is not available for a given compound, then a resynthesis of the desired compound is undertaken.

One important issue to consider is that many times hits from screening solutions which yielded >95% purity by LC/MS and nuclear magnetic resonance (NMR) failed to confirm activity upon resynthesis. This can be caused by small nuisance impurities present in the sample, which inhibit the target nonspecifically. This information should be noted in the database for future reference.

This QC topic is a very controversial one and there is not a clear response yet to questions such as what the best conditions for storing compounds are, how often should samples be QCed (only when showing up as hits or in a regular schedule?), should all file compounds be QCed before inclusion into the HTS collection, what should be the minimum purity for a compound to be maintained in the screening solution collection, and how practical is it to continually QC and remove bad compounds that are part of the HTS collection? These and other questions do not yet have clear answers, but our opinion is that all the compounds should be QCed prior to inclusion into the HTS collection, that all hits should also be analyzed, and that a regularly scheduled QC of all the compounds would be ideal, even though this creates an extra load of work. These results would be very useful in the medium term to define which are the best storage conditions and to define patterns of instability based on the structure of the compounds, so that shelf life could be assigned based on those data. Once a compound does not pass the QC criteria, ideally it should be removed from the collection or flagged in the database.

Another important consideration in the management of a compound collection is that all liquid handlers and the informatic management systems should be QCed periodically in order to ensure that the materials provided to HTS are always in the requested amount and concentration. The system should provide correct locations and remaining amounts for samples and the liquid handlers should dispense the right amounts in the right wells or tubes. The QC of the informatic systems is inherent to the process of retrieving samples to be assayed.

4.2. QC of Instruments

A process has been developed by us for the QC of the instruments (*3*). In summary, a standard operating procedure was used for liquid handling quality control (LHQC) that has enabled us to evaluate liquid handler performance on two levels. The first level provides for routine daily testing on existing instrumentation while the second level allows for evaluation of new products available in the market as candidates for our HTS process. In practice, prior to the dispensement of compounds onto assay plates, three dye plates are run according to established guidelines. An Excel template has been created to help in the analysis of the results. In order to pass this test, the results from the three plates will have to comply with all the following rules:

- Systematic errors: not acceptable if all three plates have the same well empty.
- Nonsystematic errors (total number of unacceptable errors in the three plates).
  ♦ Overdispensement
    – Assay sensitive to DMSO: <1% wells with >50% extra volume dispensed with respect to the average.
    – Assay nonsensitive to DMSO: <1% wells with >100% extra volume dispensed with respect to the average.
  ♦ Underdispensement
    – <1% wells with <50% volume dispensed with respect to the average.
    – <0.5% wells with <10% volume dispensed with respect to the average.
- Accuracy: every plate should have as average the expected volume of solution ± 20%.
- Precision: every plate should show an overall CV<10% for volumes >200 nL and <20% for volumes <200 nL.

5. Summary

The increasing size of the collections used for drug-discovery purposes has demanded both hardware and software automation of compound management in order to cope with the increasing demands of HTS. Splitting the collection into a number of copies in different formats is a desirable approach to keep a balance between rapid response to the demands and best storage conditions. Flexibility to different assay configurations can be provided with the appropriate selection of liquid handlers, and the informatic management systems should be accessible to keep track of the samples and link them to a variety of information that can help interpret HTS data. In this respect, QC data on the compounds and quality checks of the equipment used are highly desirable. It is also prudent for a large organization with different research sites to have a unified database and compatible plate format and concentration in order to be able to exchange samples and share screening results. The accomplishment of all the previous requirements is the only way to ensure an efficient and effective compound library management.

References

1 Gosnell, P. A., Hilton, A. D., Anderson, L. M., Wilkins, L., and Janzen, W. P. (1997) Compound library management in high throughput screening. *J. of Biomol. Screening* **2,** 99–102.

2. Kim, S. S., Gong, Y. D., and Yoo, S. (2000) Chemical Library Management. *Korean J. Med. Chem.* **10**, 22–38.
3. Taylor, P. B., Ashman, S., Bond, B. C., Hertzberg, R. P., Kubala, S. M., Macarron, R., et al. (2000) A Standard Operating Procedure for Assessing Liquid Handler Performance in HTS. Society for Biomolecular Screening, 6th Annual Convention and Exhibition, Vancouver, British Columbia, Canada, September 6–9.

Appendix

In this appendix some information about existing equipment is described with references to the vendors web pages when available.

1. Haywain. Compounds are being weighed manually in most organizations due the impracticability of handling different physical form of the solids. The Automation Partnership has the Haywain™ module that takes racks of dry powders in vials and weighs 0.1–3 mg accurately into vials to weigh free-flowing dry powder. Web address: http://www.autoprt.co.uk
2. Liquid-dispensing units.
    a. Multidrop. This is a rapid dispensing system very well suited for the quick dispensation of buffer onto plates. It provides a great throughput with good levels of accuracy. Web address: http://www.labsystems.fi/products/dispensers/index.htm
    b. Tomtec's Quadra: There are a number of different models in the market able to dispense from 96–1536 wells. When equipped with a low volume head, it is able to dispense down to 0.5 µL with great accuracy. It is also possible to integrate stackers for the automatic feeding of the machine. Web address: http://www.tomtec.com/Pages/products.html
    c. Robbins' Hydra and Tango: These machines are very well-suited for the dispensation of very low volumes (50 nL) and have 384–1536 reformatting capacity. The difference between the Tango and the Hydra is that the former has more deck positions to accommodate a larger number of plates. The system has been fitted with sensors to avoid mispositioning of the plates and with flexible needles to avoid replacement when any crash occurs. Web address: http://www.tomtec.com/Pages/products.html
    d. CCS/Packard's PlateTrack: The PlateTrak is an automated microplate processing system with stackers that in a single platform can accommodate plate replication (96 to 96, 384 to 384) and reformatting (4 × 96 to 384 and 4 × 384 to 1536) with acceptable CVs dispensing 0.5 µL to dry plate. The bi-directional conveyor provides secure microplate handling, accurate dispensing and efficient automation in configuration from 4–16 modules. Web Address: http://www.ccspackard.com
    e. Tecan's Genesis. This is a very well-known piece of equipment that is able to provide great flexibility in the reformatting process due to its cherry picking capability and its ability to recognize a great number of containers from flasks to plates and vials. It is fully programmable so any mapping can be achieved.

When equipped with piezo tips it can dispense very low volumes. Web address: http://www.tecan.com/index_tecan.htm

   f. Beckman's BIOMEK2000: Also a pretty standard piece of equipment that shares many of the functions of the Genesis. Web address: http://www.beckman.com/ Beckman/biorsrch/prodinfo/automated_solutions/biomek2k.asp

3. Integrator systems.

   a. Hudson's Plate crane. Web address: http://www.hudsoncontrol.com/products/ platecrane.htm

   b. Tecan's Twister. Web address: http://www.tecan.com/tec_main_twister.htm These two systems are able to move plates to given positions and greatly help to make process run unattended.

4. Middle-size store and liquid-handlers systems.

   a. Tecan's Molbank: This system integrates an automated storage system able to automatically retrieve plates and boxes stored at the user's defined conditions. It is linked to a Genesis system so it can create plates directly without human intervention. It is ideally suited for small collections. Web address: http://www.tecan.com/index_tecan.htm

8

Compound Library Management

An Overview of an Automated System

Wilma W. Keighley and Terry P. Wood

1. Introduction

The Automated Liquid Sample Bank (ALSB) is a key component of our strategy to increase drug-discovery productivity and to reduce manning requirements wherever possible.

1.1. Need for Automation in Sample Supply

Discovery management had set a challenging target for growth in candidate generation, and in order to achieve this, a coordinated strategy to increase our lead-seeking capabilities was developed. This included significant investments in combinatorial chemistry, both internally, and externally with Arqule, in order to enrich our files with thousands of drug-like molecules amenable to combinatorial follow-up. As a result of this, the then-current compound file was expected to increase by some 50% by end 2000 and it was essential that these compounds be exposed to as many of our lead seeking targets as possible. A parallel initiative, involving collaborations with Aurora and Evotec, will increase the annual number of high-throughput screens (HTS) run.

This plan implies an enormous increase in sample handling and throughput to meet the large increase in the number of HTS to be run against a growing number of biological targets, and the increase in the size of the file against which they would be run. Our ability to dispense samples for test on the scale required to support this effort was far beyond our existing manual capabilities. Our system for sample dispensation was a mixture of manual and semi-automated effort: labor intensive and prone to human error. Since our existing liquid store was contained in deep well microtiter plates, follow up of actives

From: *Methods in Molecular Biology, vol. 190: High Throughput Screening: Methods and Protocols*
Edited by: W. P. Janzen © Humana Press Inc., Totowa, NJ

required manual handling of large numbers of compounds to access the few required and meant that recourse to dry samples was the only solution for the compilation of a targeted subset, which was impractical for sets larger than several thousand compounds. If manning resource for sample preparation was not to become excessive (and we estimated that an increase of 10 FTEs would be required to meet the predicted requirements), or sample provision to prove a bottleneck in the process, the requirement for automation of the storage and dispensing process was clear.

1.2. A Secure Store

The composition of our drug file was also changing. Where once dry sample had been the major storage form for the file, increasingly high-speed chemistry was producing many compounds but in smaller quantities, such that weighing and dispensing from a dry store was not viable. The only source of the majority of our compound file soon would be from a liquid stock and it was essential that this could be securely stored and efficiently used.

1.3. Requirements of the System

Projections of the likely storage requirements, needs of HTS, and follow-up, led to a specification of an ALSB) that would have an initial capacity to store up to approx 2.8 million samples, would deliver up to 44,000 compounds per day for screening, and could support our HTS initiatives for at least seven years (specification fixed in 1997). By streamlining sample provision, ALSB was expected to make a significant impact on the number of HTS-derived CANs (compounds submitted for development) in our portfolio, and hence increase our overall productivity. ALSB would also keep us at the forefront in exploiting high-speed technologies and would provide the first step in developing a worldwide Pfizer strategy for dispensing screening samples.

The ALSB was designed to store all compounds as liquid samples at –20°C, with robotic retrieval and distribution to a range of screens via computer control. Compounds are stored individually in tubes, held in rack arrays, such that single tubes or an entire rack can be selected. Therefore HTS sets can be compiled quickly by extracting and sampling from entire racks, while thousands of samples can be assembled for screening in any order, individually, or as structurally related families, by tube-wise selection, almost 100 times faster than the existing system. Moreover, since compounds are stored in individual tubes, retrieval of active samples for follow-up of HTS is much more efficient than manual operation, that relies on retrieving and thawing entire deep-well plates. Importantly, the database of compound inventory usage and biological activity for all samples would be integrated into central information technology (IT) systems such as DISCUS (our global screening database), for rapid and reliable dissemination of information. ALSB would also be integrated with in-house compound ordering and experiment creation and analysis software to provide a smooth workflow for the scientist with a strong audit trail for compound and test result. As part of a world-wide strategy for global compound ordering and management ALSB can also be used to furnish those samples not available locally to Pfizer Global R & D centers in the USA, Europe, and Japan.

2. The Manufacture and the Design

2.1. The Idea

Once the case for an ALSB had been made (albeit not at this stage approved), the team produced a summary specification of how we saw the final product. The key goals of the system were that it should:

- Maintain a bank of samples.
- Maintain an inventory of stored samples.
- Accept orders for samples and schedule preparation.
- Prepare ordered samples by transferring the required volume from the stocks held in the bank to mother plates. If required, dilute the mother plates and produce (multiple) daughter plates.
- Interface with existing equipment and software.
- Achieve critical success factors that would assure controlled and reliable operation.
- Be a commercially realistic package both for Pfizer and for the vendor.

As we were planning to use this specification as the basis for the document that would be sent out to potential suppliers of the system, we were very careful to avoid indicating possible solutions to the goals listed previously. In this way we hoped to encourage companies to identify creative solutions rather than to redevelop our preconceived ideas.

2.2. The Tendering Process

The user requirements document was distributed to 20 companies, in both Europe and North America, together with a letter inviting the submission of tenders to design, build, and install an ALSB at the Sandwich, UK, Pfizer site. Of these only six companies were prepared to undertake the complete project, several others indicated a desire to involve themselves as subcontractors to the main contractor.

A working party involving key members of Pfizer's chemistry, biology, IT, and engineering departments was commissioned to review in detail the design-specification documents of those companies offering complete solutions. The outcome of this working party was to identify a short list of three companies. Upon notification, the three companies were invited to Sandwich to present their solution to Pfizer's ALSB requirement, and demonstrate that they were competent to undertake a project of such magnitude.

In the interim period between notification and presentation, representatives from Pfizer accepted invitations to the production facilities of each company to inspect projects in development and to the sites of previous customers who where willing to demonstrate already completed projects. In addition, Pfizer legal and financial teams investigated the viability and credibility of each of the three candidate companies.

After on-site presentations from each of the three competing companies, there followed an intensive series of internal meetings at which the case of each was minutely examined. Not surprisingly, the solution offered to the problem by each of the tendering companies was quite different in concept, though certain basic threads ran through each solution: frozen storage, single rather than multiple sample copies, tube based system, etc. For a variety of reasons, including the quality of their engineering and their reputation built on the large-scale products they had supplied to other customers, Pfizer selected the tender of RTS Thurnall (then Thurnall plc) and requested that they begin preparing a detailed proposal of how they would achieve the project objectives.

2.3. From Idea to Design

One of the more difficult aspects of the ALSB project was communication of concepts and ideas. A team of biologists and chemists had conceived how a system might automatically provide samples for biological testing. This scientific concept now had to be translated into terms that would allow a team of hardware and software engineers to identify the technical solution. The Functional Design Specification, a close look at each functional element in each area of the system, was based on a mutually agreed System Design Concept, which gave a clear description of the system input and outputs. The preparation of these documents required several hundred man-hours of discussion and debate, much of which concerned the appreciation of the relevant 'business' of each other's industries. We learned from this exercise that it is virtually impossible to explain points in too much detail. We realized, too late in some cases, that as HTS specialists, we had thought that there was only one sensible way of doing some things; however, it was wrong to assume that an engineer would have the same understanding as a biologist. From an engineer's viewpoint, alternative methods were perfectly logical, but could have caused great practical problems for the biologists.

3. Development and Building – What, Why, and How?

For reasons of compound stability, we elected that samples should be stored in 100% dimethyl sulphoxide (DMSO) at $-20°C$. In addition the system should prepare daughter plates for screening (a 'daughter' plate being defined as the screen ready plate derived by dilution from an intermediate 'mother' plate, which is derived by dilution from the 4 mM source stored in the ALSB), and that these daughter plates should be prepared in as timely a manner as possible. Therefore, at the highest level, the ALSB was to consist of a frozen store, a station in which to thaw the samples, and liquid handling robotics, all connected by a transport system. **Figure 1** shows the final layout of the system.

An attractive feature of the RTS Thurnall solution was the use of tried and tested components throughout the system. For example the Flexlink conveyor system (Flexlink Systems Ltd., Milton Keynes, UK) connecting the various parts of the ALSB is identical to that found in hundreds of factories throughout the world. Again, samples were to be stored in vertical paternoster carousels, which are widely used in warehouses and stores in many industries. The principle behind this approach was to build reliability into the system at the planning stage.

3.1. Cold Store

The cold store is a 500 m^3 room maintained at –20°C. This room houses the samples, held in racks of 90 tubes, together with about 18 tons of plant and robotics. Forty-three racks are held on each storage tray, which are held in banks of 3 at 60 levels on each of 4 Paternoster storage carousels. Multiplying up, $90 \times 43 \times 3 \times 60 \times 4$ gives the capacity of the system: in excess of 2.7 million samples. Following an order, the carousel level containing the sample will rotate to a preset position where one of 12 tray-pulling robots will pull the entire tray of 43 racks out of the carousel. The picking mechanism of one of the twin overhead gantry robots (one robot serving 2 carousels) will then select either an individual tube from a rack, or the entire rack of samples, depending upon the order makeup. These gantry robots weigh approximately one ton, are around 3 meters long, and, over an operating envelope of 9 sq. m., can position with an accuracy of 1 tenth of a millimeter. Individual tubes are placed into a transport rack, or entire racks are selected by the robots and the racks of tubes, identified by bar code, are placed on the cold-store outfeed conveyor and transported to the to the defrost oven.

3.2. Defrost Station

Since samples in 100% DMSO at –20°C will certainly be solid, prior to aspiration the samples are gently thawed into the liquid state in the defrost station. Racks of samples are transferred from the Input/Output port connecting the defrost station with the cold store, to the next available shelf of a Carbolite Paternoster oven (Carbolite Furnaces Ltd., Sheffield, UK) contained in the defrost station. After a pre-set time, the rack of samples, now thawed, is

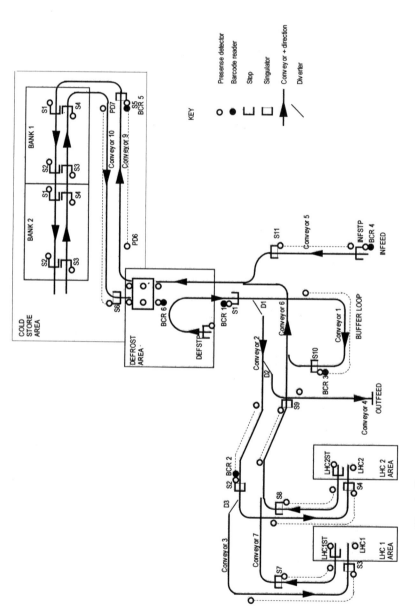

Fig. 1. Compound library management – an overview of an automated system.

picked and placed on the conveyor leading into the laboratory environment of the ALSB. The operating temperature of the oven, and the time samples are contained within it have been selected to minimize thermal exposure, while ensuring the entire rack of frozen samples are completely thawed. In addition, the defrost station atmosphere is maintained at 15% relative humidity to reduce ingress of water into the cold-store environment.

Samples being returned to storage bypass the oven and are carried straight back into the cold store, passing under a high velocity air stream to evaporate any post liquid-handling micro-droplets that might possibly adhere to the top of the septum seal of the tubes.

3.3. Liquid-Handling Cells

The ALSB system has twin liquid handling cells in which the samples are aspirated, diluted, and dispensed into the format specified in the originating order. The hardware configuration of each cell is identical, and is shown in **Fig. 2**. Selection of which liquid handling cell a sample rack is sent to is made by the system software with priority to keep samples from the same order together. If required, it is possible to manually override the system selection.

Incoming racks of tubes are picked up by a 6-axis Stäubli robotic arm (Stäubli Unimation Ltd., Telford, UK) that traverses the length of the cell. As part of the failsafe design, status checks occur at all stages, and the initial operation of the Stäubli robot is to run the rack of tubes it has picked past the on-board barcode reader to ensure the samples are those specified at this stage of the order process. The rack is placed on one of nine positions on twin platens designed to locate in the operating envelope of a Tecan Genesis robotic sample processor (Tecan UK, Reading, UK). This twin platen arrangement allows the Genesis to work on the contents of one platen while the Stäubli robot unloads or loads the second platen. Dilution algorithm software calculates the most efficient and compound sparing aspirate-dispense protocol to achieve the delivered volume, compound concentration and DMSO concentration, in the output plates specified in the original order.

The Stäubli robot collects the appropriate labware from infeed stack locations, checking each selection by scanning its type identifying bar code. Prior to liquid handling, the system sprays the order information on a blank label on the final destination (daughter) plate. Once all labware is assembled the platen retracts and the Genesis probes pierce the tube septa to aspirate the sample. All destination racks are open but since the source tubes are sealed the probes are designed with an outer jacket open to the atmosphere to equalize pressure each side of the sample tube.

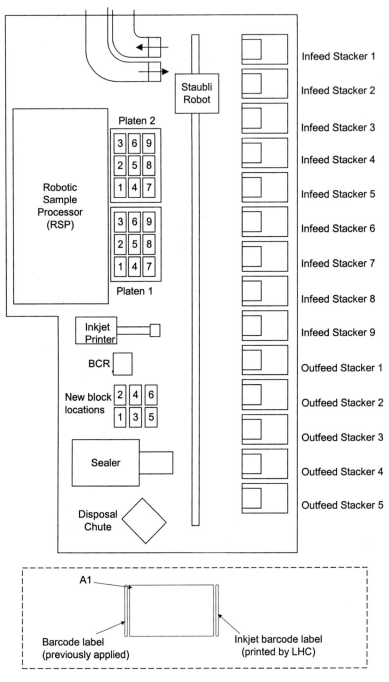

Fig. 2. Hardware configuration of an ALSB liquid handling cell.

A further modification of the Genesis is a grid held above the tube racks through which the probes can pass. This grid prevents tubes being carried with the probes once they retract through the septa. Once all liquid handling is complete, the transport rack and tubes is placed on the outfeed conveyor loop for return to the cold store. The volume field for each tube in the database is decremented by the amount aspirated. Labware used in the order is sealed, daughter plates being delivered to the outfeed stacks, and any labware used for intermediate dilutions dropped into the disposal bin. The capacity of each liquid-handling cell allows up to 1200 microplates to be available at one time, together with an outfeed capacity of 700 plates.

3.4. Transport System

The three major components of the ALSB—cold store, defrost station, and liquid-handling cells—are connected by a series of 10 Flexlink conveyor systems. In order to optimize the use of space, the conveyors are on two levels, the upper being outfeed and the lower level for infeed, relative to the cold store. Components situated along the transport system include:

- Barcode readers to confirm the correct identity of each rack at critical points in the system.
- Diverters, which direct sample racks along the selected path when there is a junction point, e.g., to divert to either of the liquid-handling cells.
- Singulators, which allow only one rack at a time to feed into certain areas, such as the pickup point between the cold store and defrost station.
- Presence Detectors, which pick up a signal from a downstream unit that a rack is in transit, and will alert the operator should the correct labware not be detected within a certain time period.
- Software-controlled retractable stops prevent buffer loops and the defrost station from overfilling.

With safety a key consideration in the ALSB, all drive wheels and conveyor stub ends are guarded, and the track itself is contained within a series of hinged Perspex covers, which, once the relevant conveyor section is halted, can be lifted for cleaning and maintenance. Emergency stop buttons are widely distributed across the system.

3.5. Controlling Software

The software hierarchy of the ALSB is shown in **Fig. 3**.

The Sun Ultra server (Sun Microsystems Inc., Palo Alto, CA) operates using the Solaris UNIX platform, with external disc storage comprising twinned disc sets operating in RAID 0+1 mode and an Oracle RDBS (Oracle Corp., Redwood Shores, CA) providing data storage.

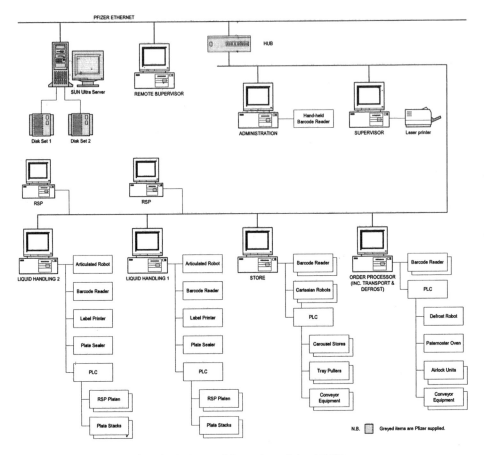

Fig. 3. Software hierarchy of the ALSB.

The controlling and processing computers, and the main ALSB database server, are networked using TCP/IP communications over an Ethernet based Local Area Network (LAN). A bridge connects this LAN to the Pfizer network.

Each 'Application Server' is dedicated to a particular major component of the ALSB, and the status of each these component can be monitored by accessing the relevant server PC. In normal use, these PCs remain locked in the service panels, but should an alarm or a need for maintenance arise, each component can be switched to manual control in order to diagnose and usually rectify the fault.

The Administrator Terminal is the hub of the ALSB from which an order's status can be checked, database queries made, and new samples entered. The administration system is provided with a Graphical User Interface (GUI), which allows the operator to menu select the various programs that manage the ALSB inventory. Data processing and verification are performed by this system against the ALSB database, and the external Pfizer corporate database, for every administration order. A hand-held barcode scanner aids the identification of specified blocks for entry or replacement. Within the program the operator is provided with selection lists as a guide to performing other transactions based upon predefined criteria for the order type.

A further PC is dedicated to System Control and Data Acquisition (SCADA) software. SCADA supplies a schematic overview of the ALSB in its entirety, and allows the operator a real time snapshot of all the system's components, and the position of any sample racks currently being used in an order. SCADA also interfaces with the Pfizer-specific Building and Environmental Management System (BEMS) and alerts an operator should an alarm situation occur at any time during 24/7 operation.

3.6. Compound Ordering Software

The Order Processor validates orders submitted to the ALSB database and performs short-term scheduling of these orders. This PC processes and schedules orders issued from the Administration System and constantly monitors the order queues in the ALSB triggering the initiation of the next order. The Order Processor monitors and updates the status of all orders issued to the ALSB. Only the administrator is able to generate orders directly via this interface, customers of the system have two purpose built user interfaces which give access to the system; these are described in **Subheading 7.**

4. Labware
4.1. Design

At an early stage in the functional design program, Pfizer agreed with RTS Thurnall that Pfizer would take responsibility for the supply of the storage media that would contain the liquid samples in ALSB. RTS Thurnall did, however, supply specifications as to required size and tolerance of each component. As the labware would be used across the total operating temperature range of the system, these tolerances turned out to be more difficult to achieve than originally imagined. At its most basic, the storage medium specified required a microtiter formatted rack bar-coded at one end, with various slots and holes in the body of the rack to allow robotic grippers to operate, air to circulate, and for the rack to locate, without slippage, on a storage tray. The rack would contain 1 mL polypropylene tubes, each carrying a unique (human readable) identifier, and sealed with a silicon-rubber septum, and conform to a maximum weight specification.

4.2. The Tubes

A tube already available from Marsh Biomedical conformed to the tube specification, and we decided to design the rest of the storage system around this tube. However, it did not carry an identifier, and although in theory tube marking was not necessary, as the software would track all tubes, we wanted the 'feel good' factor that the tubes could, if necessary, be physically identified. In practice, tube identification has proved to be an extremely useful feature. At the time we were designing the storage medium, the uniquely identifiable tubes currently on the market were not available (uniquely identified tubes now available from Integra Biosciences, Traxis® and Matrix Technologies, Trakmate®). Although several manufacturers made claim, none proved able to legibly and durably print or adhere either an electronic or human readable label on the tubes. One remaining possibility was to laser-etch a number on the side of each tube. We had practical experience that this was possible, but concerns that this might not be practical for the large numbers of tubes that we had to prepare.

The challenge was to design and build a machine to laser-etch a unique identifier on each of 1 million tubes, and to electronically associate that number with what would be the rack number and rack position of that tube. We decided that the tube number should be driven by the rack in which the tube was located, thus the tube in position A1 of Rack 1 should be numbered 1, while H12 in rack 1 would be number 96. Tubes numbers in each following rack would increment by 96, therefore it would be possible to predict a tube number by knowing its rack number and location and likewise given the tube number, its rack number and location would be a given. Our solution was to purchase the Marsh tubes already racked and to build a machine to pick up tubes, eight at a time from the source rack, pass them in front of a laser-gun etcher, and transfer the tubes to a destination rack. The laser gun was programmed to etch an incrementing number calculated from the rack number, for each tube. As the software disallowed the repetition of any number, we now had generated a set of uniquely identified tubes.

4.3. The Racks

The destination or storage racks mentioned earlier presented us with another set of challenges The ALSB design allows not only whole racks of tubes to be selected, but also individual tubes. Therefore a key factor in the rack design was that tubes could be freely pulled from, and inserted into, their storage racks over the 40°C range of operating temperature. If the surface of the rack face was not perfectly flat, the tubes would 'stick.' In addition, the holes in the rack could not be oversize otherwise the tubes would have too much lateral movement and may not lie perfectly vertical. Additionally, as we were limited on the mass of the rack, we could not use excessive material in the moulding. After much consultation with a local toolmaker, many prototypes, and reworks of the moulding tool, we finally produced a satisfactory rack. The finished product was a two-piece design with the base locating into the body of the rack. The weight was within limit and tubes could be removed and replaced freely across the specified range of temperatures. However, when the rack was used at –20°C we discovered that for approx 1 in 1000 of the units the rack base became detached from the rack body under operational conditions. There was no option but to recall the entire production run of 10,000 units and have the two components spot-welded together. After several design iterations, we now had our racks.

4.4. The Tube Septa

Each sample tube in the ALSB was to be sealed with a silicon-rubber septum, the performance specification of these septa necessarily being very stringent. Operationally, samples are aspirated from the tubes through a Tecan Genesis probe designed for septum piercing. The septa were required to remain airtight after 160 penetrations by the probe, and during that period show no sign of coring or of being pushed into the tube. We found that once the septum had been pierced for a first time, subsequent piercing tended to follow the original track through the septum. We were able capitalize on this feature by designing a funnel-shaped guide above the tube, so that probes tended to pierce in the same area of the septum each time. We also required that no biologically or chemically active substances would be leached from the septa during contact with DMSO. Again, we were fortunate to have a specialist local company who were contracted to work with us through many prototypes, until we identified the optimum material and manufacturing process to produce the septa we required. We now had all the components of the storage media. All that remained was to put them together and transfer our samples into this ALSB compatible labware.

5. Preparation of Samples
5.1. Transfer of the Legacy Set of Compounds

Samples at Pfizer are stored as both dry compounds and as presolubilized solutions, and it is from the latter bank that HTS and follow-up screening are sourced. It was this legacy set of some half-million samples that was to be transferred to the new labware. The liquid-handling challenge was daunting, and each sample had to be positively and accurately identified in its new location, and this information loaded into the ALSB database. In addition we were required to populate a sample-volume field in this database, a parameter that, for the vast majority of our legacy set, was unrecorded. All samples were stored in deep-well microtiter plates, and without a computer-legible label of content. The first task was to transfer the entire contents of each plate into the ALSB tube sets using a Quadra 96 dispenser. At each transfer, the identity of the source plate was associated with the destination ALSB tube set id using a PC networked with our corporate compound database. To ensure accuracy, we ran a two-person buddy system, with each association being checked prior to it being committed. The task was simple, but the magnitude daunting, as we had around 6000 deep-well plates to transfer.

We had made the decision to insert septa into the tubes after liquid transfer, and our research workshop designed and built a machine with a rotating cutter that removed a septum from a moulding of 96 septa and spun it into a destination tube. We later commissioned an engineering company to build two further machines based on the initial design of this ingenious prototype.

Perhaps the most difficult task was the final one of accurately estimating the volume of liquid sample in each tube, and again, reporting this to the corporate database. After much deliberation over technique, a Swedish company devised a system that picked up 8 tubes at a time, and took a real-time image of the tubes. Software measured the height between the base of the tube and the meniscus of the liquid, and knowing the tube's geometry, calculated the contained volume. In double-blind trials the device proved to be highly accurate for both clear and colored solutions. Moreover, the robotics of the system allowed volume estimation at a rate of over 1500 tubes per hour, much greater than that which could be achieved by weighing, the main alternative we had considered.

The project of designing the ALSB compatible labware, transferring our legacy sample set, assimilating the new data into corporate and ALSB databases involved a Pfizer team of over 20 engineers, scientists, and information technologists and took almost two years to complete. Despite the demands made on sample supply logistics by the transfer process, during that time it was necessary and indeed we were still able to resource our entire ongoing battery of high throughput and follow up screening programs.

5.2. Methods for New Samples

During the period of legacy sample transfer, our synthetic chemistry and sample-acquisition programs were still supplying samples for file enrichment. Together with an external software house we developed a liquid-handling program that manipulated mass and molecular-weight parameters from flat files to solubilize new samples to an exact molarity. The program then transfers a recorded volume to a rack of ALSB tubes that are sealed and entered into the system. Solid-sample solubilization, distribution, and database update is now a fully automated, continuous process requiring very little operator intervention. Acquired liquid samples simply require transfer to ALSB labware and an electronic association of the incoming sample details with the destination ALSB rack identifier.

6. Milestones in the Project

6.1. Acceptance Testing: The Test Document

Jointly with RTS Thurnall, a battery of tests designed to comprehensively examine all aspects of the ALSB's function, operation, and performance were devised. This Acceptance Test Script (ATS) was used as a common testing scenario to ensure that the machine performed to specification, to the satisfaction of both RTS Thurnall and Pfizer, after factory build and again following subsequent site installation.

The ATS comprised 7 main sections and included a total of 97 discrete tests. These sections and what they contained are summarized in **Table 1**.

In order to operate the tests, a purpose-specific database of sample information and order types was designed, created, and loaded into the ALSB: together with hundreds of racks containing dummy samples.

6.2. IFAT (Internal Factory Acceptance Test)

The final stage of the build program at RTS Thurnall's Manchester factory was to ensure the machine performed in accordance with the functional design specification to which it was built, and that the system design would in fact deliver when translated from concept to actual process. This initial stage of acceptance testing, performed by RTS Thurnall staff, inevitably identified a number of hardware and software problems requiring system modifications. These problems, together with a diagnosis of the root cause, and the eventual solutions, were recorded and satisfactory resolution of all System Trouble Notes (STNs) became a condition of system acceptance.

After several weeks testing, RTS Thurnall indicated that IFAT had been satisfactorily completed, and invited a team from Pfizer to rerun the battery of test defined in the ATS.

6.3. CFAT (Customer Factory Acceptance Test)

A team of four Pfizer scientists, with an expertise covering liquid handling, biological screening, and information technology, worked together with a team of mechanical and software engineers from RTS Thurnall to conduct CFAT. The combined test team spent 2 wk during April 1999, working 15 h per day,

Table 1
Acceptance Test Script Scope

Administrator form operation	Functionality of all GUI forms that allow the administrator to set orders.
Administrator transactions	Testing of all sample withdrawal, replacement, and replenishment capabilities described in the specification.
Daughter plate orders	Ensure the system delivers all per missible variations of daughter-plate format.
Access procedures	The various elements within the ALSB must be accessible, but only when the system is in a safe condition.
Replenishment of consumable items	Demonstration that all consumable storage modules are accessible, operable, and give suitable alerts when running low.
Alarm conditions and recovery from failure	Simulation of a wide range of hard-ware, software, and service failures, to demonstrate that the equipment fails safe and the system is recoverable.
Performance testing	Does the system deliver its required output within the time frames specified.

conducting an identical set of tests to those performed at IFAT. This testing culminated in acceptance of the system performance by Pfizer. The work was very demanding, but the camaraderie between the two teams was tremendous, which further cemented the strong relationship that had been built up between the two companies during design and development, and which proved to be a great asset in the final stages of the project.

With the customer factory acceptance testing complete, the onus was now on RTS Thurnall to dismantle the equipment, ship it to Pfizer's Sandwich site, and then begin a program of installation and commissioning. RTS Thurnall indicated that they were ready for the final test phase to commence in December 1999.

6.4. SAT (Site Acceptance Test)

The Pfizer team now prepared to run the ATS for the third time. The major difference between CFAT and SAT was that the cold store was now at its operating temperature of –20°C, whereas during factory testing the store had been at room temperature. This made a big difference to the timing of various performance tests, as each test involving liquid handling had to be preceded by a 3-h thawing cycle. Not only did Pfizer require all 97 tests be successfully completed, they also insisted that all STNs raised during the test and commissioning periods—a total of 437—be satisfactorily resolved.

On January 20, 2000, almost five years to the day the original concept document had been presented to senior management, Pfizer formally accepted delivery of the ALSB.

As a stand-alone system, ALSB worked, but it was still necessary to complete the integration of ALSB with Pfizer software packages DISCUS, ECADA, and IMSO, without which ALSB could not be used.

6.5. PINT (Pfizer Integration)

Integration testing was conducted using test instances of the Pfizer databases. DISCUS (Discovery Universal Server), which holds the compound inventory; ECADA (Experiment Creation and Data Analysis), which manages HTS data; and the compound ordering application IMSO (Inventory Management and Sample Ordering), which provides both a direct user interface for ALSB plus an interface to connect HTS experiment creation with ordering from ALSB. Details of the connectivity of these applications are shown in **Fig. 4**. For the purposes of testing, these databases were populated with dummy data to ensure that incompatibilities could be identified and resolved before interfacing ALSB with the live applications and databases. This stage in the implementation of ALSB was not made easier by being conducted across the Y2K changeover period, which meant double testing in many cases and scarcity of IT resource to resolve problems. Good planning did, however, pay dividends and this part of the testing procedure was completed successfully on schedule.

7. User Interfaces

Introduction of the ALSB at Sandwich not only meant having a new repository for liquid samples, and major changes in the working practises of the liquid-handling team, it also meant substantial changes for the screening scientists who would be the customers of ALSB. Prior to automation of sample selection and preparation, scientists had ordered their samples by a variety of means including telephone, e-mail, and electronic ordering. Automation of the

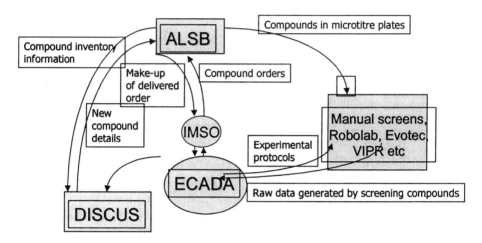

Fig. 4. Compound library management – an overview of an automated system.

task meant that all ordering had to become electronic, a substantial change for users. Luckily, there were also substantial benefits to the users of this new system with which to sweeten the change.

Previously, if users required samples for HTS, they could expect to have to give several weeks notice to the liquid-handling team in order that their samples would be ready when required; ALSB means that samples are available much faster. Users requiring bespoke selection of compounds had no alternative but to have these weighed as dry samples to order by our Compound Control Centre and expect to wait several months should the selected set be more than a few thousand compounds; again ALSB is much faster. To allow users to gain full benefit of the capabilities of ALSB, we realized it was essential to give them efficient and user-friendly ordering tools as their interface with the system. Two applications, which have been designed and built in-house, are available to users to select and order their samples, each with a specific range of functionality.

7.1. IMSO (Inventory Management and Sample Ordering)

IMSO is our basic ordering application that handles both solid and liquid compound requests as well as stores orders for chemicals. Some of the functionality of IMSO is not directly relevant to the ALSB, but it does provide a common front end for selection of both dry and liquid samples for test. Within IMSO, users can:

- Select individual compounds or racks of compounds based on the compound number or the rack name (all racks of compounds have logical prefixes denoting specific 'sources' of compound).

- Conduct substructure searches (IMSO uses the structural searching powers of MDL's ISIS (MDL Information Systems Inc., San Leandru, CA) and build a selection on the basis of the search.
- IMSO can import a text-file of compound numbers so that a selection compiled by any other means can be submitted as an order to ALSB.

When selections of individual compounds are submitted, IMSO checks the ALSB location of each compound in the selection. If the majority of compounds on a rack are selected by an order, IMSO will suggest to the user that the whole rack is supplied (which is a more efficient operation for the robotics) but the user can decline if they so choose. Within IMSO, the user selects the plate type in which they want to receive their samples (from a selection available within ALSB), the concentration of compound and the % DMSO which they require, and the volume of solution required. It is the users' responsibility to take account of any further dilutions, etc., to which their samples will be subject and they must select the volume and concentration required accordingly.

7.2. ECADA (Experiment Creation and Data Analysis)

ECADA is our main data tracking and analysis tool for in vitro screening. Primarily designed to handle HTS, ECADA also serves lower throughput projects if the in vitro assay records similar parameters to a HTS (e.g., % compound effect at a range of, or a single, concentration). Its primary purpose is to support the screening process and, as such, it handles setting up of screens and experiments within those screens, ordering the compounds that will be used in these experiments and checking on the status of compound orders. ECADA captures the raw data generated by the experiments, assists the user to check the quality of the data, and analyse and validate the data for transfer to the corporate database.

Via ECADA scientists can:

- Select compounds for screening by compound number, by plate identifier or by compound set (for example compounds targeted to specific target types, or sets coming from specific locations).
- In cases where the number of compounds selected cannot conveniently be screened in one day, ECADA will schedule experiments at rates selected by the experimenter and place orders against ALSB for just in time delivery.
- ECADA can import text files to create an order list.
- Can automatically create a new ALSB order based on the active compounds from a previous experiment.

Because ALSB selects compounds within an order in the most efficient picking order, ECADA has to construct the experiment to match the order sequence of compounds supplied by ALSB. All this is transparent to the user.

7.3. Provision for Automated Systems as Customer

The customer of the ALSB output is not always a screening scientist. Many of our HTS screens are now run on fully automated systems such as Robolab and Beckman-Sagian linear tracks and Evotec uHTS devices. In some cases, the output from ALSB requires reformatting before delivery to the scientist and, here too, the recipient of the ALSB output plate is a robotic system. All output plates from ALSB bear a human readable label printed directly onto the plates at time of liquid handling in ALSB. This label gives details of the number of plates in the order and sequence of the individual plate, plus recipient's name, etc. The same information is also held in a barcode printed on the label again at liquid handling which the other automated devices can read. The barcode gives information about what should happen to this plate and which compounds it contains, so, for example, should plates get out of sequence during running of the assay, the data will still be associated with the correct compound via the barcode check. Reformatting systems could also apply various dilution or reformatting regimes to intermediate plates arriving from ALSB according to details on each barcode (*see* **Subheading 8.2.**). However, selection of a bar-coding symbology is not a trivial detail in integrating systems one with another. Code EAN 128 was selected as the barcode system which ALSB would utilize and this has meant that we have preferred to have the other elements of our automation (screening robotic, etc.) making use of the same system. On occasion, this has proved to be less simple than one might expect and, with hindsight, selection of a symbology system in more common use in the pharmaceutical industry would have been preferred.

8. Capacity

8.1. Input and Output Metrics

As described in **Subheading 3.** this first stage of ALSB has a capacity of greater than 2.7 million samples. We estimated this capacity to be sufficient until at least 2004 at current rate of sample acquisition (although since this estimate the merger of Pfizer and Warner Lambert has taken place and is likely to demand a re-estimate). The design of the system allows for incorporation of a second cold store at a later date, with space for up to 4 more paternosters that would increase capacity to 5.6 million individual samples.

Our output requirements for ALSB were based on estimated screening requirements over the next five years and, necessarily, involved a lot of best guesses. Does anything change so fast as HTS technology? Central to our philosophy was the idea that ALSB should be kept simple, should not be constantly altered to support each new requirement, but rather that we would obtain speed from a simple ALSB output and flexibility from ancillary systems that could modify that initial output. Thus, ALSB stores compounds in a 96-place array, and produces output in this same array, though the majority of our screening currently demands a 384 array. As stated previously, ALSB operates in two modes: rack-based (where the customer requires all, or nearly all, of the compounds in a rack) or tube-based (where a customized selection of compounds for screening from a wide range of racks is made). A conservative estimate of ALSB output rate for rack-based orders is 600 racks per day (limited generally by liquid-handling rate) and for tube-based orders is 6000 tubes per day (limited by tube-picking robotics). Most days a mix of tube- and rack-based orders results thus maximizing the usage of both liquid handling and robotic tube picking. We judged these to be adequate throughput rates to satisfy screening at least until 2005. This is based on likely number and rate of screens to be run, likely number of compounds to be screened, which leads to an estimate of rack-based orders. In addition, the likely follow-up rate per HTS and potential use of targeted subsets, etc., leads to estimates of tube-based requirements. Our usage strategy is also designed to be compound sparing. Although there are liquid-handling devices on the market that can aspirate and dispense much smaller volumes than 5 μL, most would be unable to pierce the re-sealable caps that close our tubes.

Additionally we chose to keep this as our lowest aspirate volume via the Tecan Genesis robots that form the liquid-handling system for ALSB because, in our experience, Genesis liquid handlers offer reliability, accuracy, and precision at the 5 μL level and this is all important in a 24×7 walkaway system. In the case of most HTS, 5 μL of 4 mM compound, however diluted, will be in vast excess to the requirements of the screen and hence wasteful of compound. Currently, the vast majority of our HTS utilise the same screening set of compounds, therefore it is possible to use the same intermediate plates (at, say, 200 μM) to supply multiple HTS at primary screen level with ALSB being used to restock these intermediate plates as required.

8.2. Supporting Systems

Plate replication, (to produce many HTS sets from one ALSB output plate) is handled by 96/384 and 384/384 liquid-handling systems and allows us to make full use of the ALSB output while retaining flexibility over dilution buffer, % DMSO, and final assay concentration to suit the individual screen. Our main workhorse for this type of work is the Matrix Platemate (in Europe now marketed as CyBi-well from CyBio) although we also use Tomtec Quadra and Packard Platetrak systems for similar tasks. At present, operators take the output from ALSB and, from knowledge of the contents of the output and knowledge of the required HTS input plate, program the Platemate to transfer the appropriate volume of compound, plus correct diluent to the target plate(s). To remove the potential for human error in this process, we are developing a system whereby the Platemate, following barcode reading, will automatically select the appropriate liquid-handling program. The selection is being based on the output and target information which has been written to database tables by ALSB (output information) and by ECADA (target information).

An additional customer for ALSB output is our Evotec uHTS system. This screening system consists of two parts, Mitona, which reformats 96- or 384-well plates into Evotec format nanocarriers (2280 well, 1536 of which are compound containing), and Scarina, which carries out the HTS. The output of ALSB can go directly into Mitona where each nanocarrier is compiled from the contents of sixteen, 96-well microtiter plates. Additionally, it is possible to make replicate copies of each nanocarrier (this is the most efficient way in terms of both speed and compound usage of preparing a large number of plates with Mitona), which act as a source of screening plates for future assays.

In both examples, one production of a full HTS file by ALSB can supply many complete primary HTS.

9. Changing Processes: Need for Confidence

Before our ALSB was completed and open for use, we realized that we needed to educate our scientists to these new ways of working, which would be necessary in order to take full advantage of what ALSB has to offer. Scientists who had always used dry compound and had solubilized and diluted their own samples would now be relying on the fidelity of a sample produced by an automated system. Further, scientists had to be convinced that a compound stored long-term, in 100% DMSO, at −20°C, which had possibly been through several freeze-thaw cycles, was as good as the freshly weighed sample they might previously have received. We tried to address this challenge in a number of ways.

9.1. Publicity

Prior to the launch of ALSB, we attended and presented at communications meetings for most of those departments that we knew would be customers of ALSB. The presentation that we developed was altered at each meeting, tailored to suit the needs of the audience. Thus, for chemists we focused on abilities to select a subset of compounds based on structural searching and on quality-control aspects, which would ensure the integrity of the chemical file. Biologists were mainly interested in how to order compounds by screening set and what assay-plate formats could be supplied. We also spent considerable effort explaining the business need for the system to our IT helpdesk, database managers, facilities managers, and mechanical engineering support—all of those people who would have an impact on the support of the system—to gain their commitment to the critical importance of this new technology.

9.2. Liquid/Solid IC$_{50}$s

Those of us working in HTS at Pfizer have been used to receiving all of our screening samples in liquid form for many years; this was the only way the rate of sample supply could be raised to meet the demands of HTS. However many of our therapeutic zone colleagues were accustomed to receiving dry sample, which they could weigh, dissolve, and dilute themselves to prepare fresh solutions as required. Comparative data was gathered using samples from liquid store and the corresponding freshly made solution from dry sample. Most of this data was produced by colleagues in HTS who were persuaded to include liquid and dry sourced samples in their IC$_{50}$ tests for follow-up to primary HTS.

In general, the data show that data from liquid and solid IC$_{50}$ are comparable to that from repeat testing, on different days, of dry samples. Also, there is no consistent trend in potency data from solid and liquid samples since approx 50% of cases showed a higher IC$_{50}$ value from dry compared with liquid samples while 50% showed the reverse. This is not to say that all samples store well at $-20°C$ in DMSO (or under any other conditions), but that, in general, this is a suitable set of storage conditions. Confirming compound fidelity using a biological endpoint limits the data to that which can be gathered for compounds with activity against a particular biological target and is an indirect measure of compound integrity. Inevitably, this set of compounds will already have some similar structural features and so may not be representative of the file as a whole. The variations of a biological assay also impinge on the data gathered, lead us to make assumptions about the reason for the biological activity, and render it less precise than we would wish. Our desire to have a direct quantitative measure of compound integrity is fulfilled using on-line LC-MS quantification of compounds from ALSB.

9.3. LC-MS Purity/Identity Checking

Pfizer's compound file, like that of most other Pharmas, is a heterogeneous collection. Historically, all compounds were stored dry, in some quantity, with a replicate liquid inventory being constructed during the last ten years, which was available alongside the dry sample. For many samples in our file, this is still the case and so comparisons by LC-MS of the two samples are possible and the integrity of the liquid sample after variable storage periods can be assessed (always assuming that the integrity of the dry sample is not in doubt).

For newer samples entering the compound file, in particular those generated by high speed chemistry, mass of sample dictates that only a liquid sample can be held, there being insufficient material generated to permit weighing and dispensing of dry sample. For these samples, LC-MS trace of the original sample is available to compare with that generated after a period of storage. Until recently, speed of analysis of samples meant that only those interesting actives from a primary screen would be subject to structural confirmation and purity check. However, newer technology, comprising reduction in size and increase in capacity, has allowed a LC-MS with sufficient throughput to permit purity checking in quantity to be installed alongside ALSB. We plan to sample a proportion of all samples ordered from ALSB on an ongoing basis allowing us to build up a purity profile of our liquid file. We shall also be sampling a representative set of compounds on a periodic basis to gauge the changes in compound integrity over time, which may allow us to build up knowledge as to structural classes that are unstable even under such storage. This structure and purity checking will also help gain the confidence of biologists and chemists alike in the integrity of liquid samples.

10. Conclusion

This brief article has tried to encapsulate over five years of work not only from a dedicated core team, but also from over a hundred other scientists, technologists, and engineers who contributed along the route from concept to reality. The project was often difficult, frequently frustrating, but never anything less than a fascinating challenge. At time of writing we have been operating ALSB for a number of months and appreciate we are still on the steep part of the learning curve of how to get the best out of the system. A meeting called shortly after the system went live, to discuss possible enhancements, produced a list of over 40 items! A valuable lesson was learned that with a project of this magnitude, you cannot expect to get it right from day one. However, the entire team is convinced that from an ALSB derived liquid sample, we can produce solid data.

Acknowledgments

We are grateful to Dr. Nick Terrett and Mr. Michael Pollard for critical reading of this manuscript.

9

Natural Products or Not? How to Screen for Natural Products in the Emerging HTS Paradigm

Susan P. Manly, Ramesh Padmanabha, and Susan E. Lowe

1. Value of Natural Products: The Screening Perspective

Natural products are undeniably the best source for diversity in chemotype for the discovery of novel therapeutics. One-third of the top selling drugs in the world are natural products or their derivatives (**Fig. 1**). Roughly 60% of the anti-tumor and anti-infective agents that are available commercially or were in late-stage clinical development from 1989–1995 are of natural products origin *(1,2)*.

Despite the success of natural products as a source for discovery, the interest in natural products as a source of new drugs has experienced highs and lows over the years. Remarkably, it has been estimated that less than 0.5% of the total microbial population in soil samples has ever been tested *(3)*. Furthermore, a similar low percentage has been tested for other types of natural products, such as plants, microbes from the ocean, and so on. The implication here is that, given the advances allowing access to these new samples, the actual diversity available from natural products has barely been tapped.

New developments that allow the cloning of genomes from "unculturable" microbes allow access to their gene products and gene operons. Use of these new genes in traditional expression systems may result in the production of unique natural products. Plant cell culture is opening up another source of practically unlimited diversity for secondary metabolites, not only those naturally found, but also through modification of the culture conditions, a whole panoply of new secondary metabolites.

Our experience is that samples derived from natural products can be successfully utilized in discovery programs, feeding surprising novelty into the pipeline. Our experience has also taught us that the identification of the active

From: *Methods in Molecular Biology, vol. 190: High Throughput Screening: Methods and Protocols*
Edited by: W. P. Janzen © Humana Press Inc., Totowa, NJ

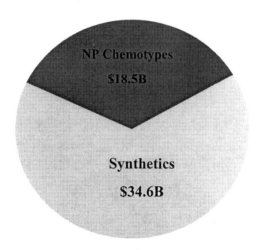

Fig. 1. 1999 Top 25 Prescription Drugs: Schematic representation of 1999's earnings for the 25 top selling prescription drugs, in billions of dollars.

principles present in the natural product samples can be facilitated up front by treatment of the samples prior to screening and by some accommodation in the screening process for the sample type, especially for crude natural product samples (**Fig. 2** and **Subheading 3.1.2.**).

In this chapter, we give details for: 1) the culturing of standard soil organisms and 2) plant preparation to produce samples with an eye toward utilizing this excellent sample source for pharmaceutical screening programs. We also include technological tips on handling the samples to speed the isolation of the active principles found in the screening portion of the discovery program. We also offer some specific, interesting examples to illustrate some of the unique challenges novel natural products offer to drug-discovery programs.

2. Discovery of Pharmacologically Relevant Natural Products from Microbial and Plant Secondary Metabolites

The approach taken in the selection of the microorganisms for investigation of secondary metabolite production is somewhat different from the criteria used for the selection of plants. Actinomycetes and fungi have historically proven to be rich producers of secondary metabolites. These organisms, commonly isolated from soil, can also be found in leaf litter, live plants, and dung. Even among microbiologists there is no consensus as to the optimal conditions for selection of soil. One view is that different microorganisms will be present in different soils because the selection pressures from different environments will lead to microorganisms differing in their physiology and metabolism. The opposite view is that every microbe is available in the back garden and there is no need to collect soil from all over the world. There are various views on how broad the taxonomic diversity of the microorganisms to be screened for secondary metabolite production should be. However, as the goal is to maximize the diversity of the secondary metabolites produced, we have found the best strategy is to include a broad variety of taxonomically diverse microorganisms.

Once the microorganisms have been selected, the cultures can be grown in either liquid or solid conditions in a variety of fermentation media. Each natural products or fermentation group has developed a variety of their own production media. Some media are very specific for the production of one secondary metabolite from a certain microorganism, which usually arises as a result of medium optimization after the active natural product has been identified. Other media are more universal, resulting in a variety of secondary metabolites being detected from taxonomically distinct microorganisms. The more universal media are used for the fermentation of microorganisms for production of secondary metabolites for HTS and are generally considered proprietary to each pharmaceutical or biotechnology company.

There are many considerations for the selection of plants as producers of valuable secondary metabolites *(4,5)*. One approach is random selection; casting the net wide and choosing plants from different taxonomic groups and different areas. An alternative method would be selective selection of plants using ethnobotanical information in which there has been local use in traditional medicine. An approach that focuses on maximum diversity of the plants would make the selection based on taxonomy, geographical location or compound structural type preferences *(4)*. A novel approach to plant selection uses the Literature Information Selection Technique (LIST), a computer-based selection method that correlates biological activity, botanical and chemotaxonomic information using the NAPRALERT® database *(5–7)*. There are many factors that can influence the type and abundance of secondary metabolites produced by plants including seasonal variations, altitude of the collection site, healthy vs diseased plants, plant age, plant part, and soil type. In addition, these variations can make reproducibility of the recollection very challenging. This can often be minimized by collecting sufficient quantities of the plant prior to extraction or by the taking of meticulous notes regarding the collection conditions.

A newer approach to maximizing the secondary metabolites produced by plants is through the use of plant cell culture. A number of companies have started to explore this area. A culture collection is compiled and then using a variety of fermentation techniques these cell cultures can be grown and the secondary metabolites produced can be evaluated for uniqueness and/or biological activity. Using this approach it is possible to produce secondary metabolites that are found in nature, as well as new compounds that would not be produced in the native habitat. Another way to modify the structure of a natural product is through the use of biotransformation.

3. Format of Natural Products as an Integral Part of a Company's Screening Deck

3.1. Crude Extracts: Advantages and Disadvantages

Traditionally microbial secondary metabolites have been screened as crude extracts in high-throughput screening (HTS). This involves growing the organism under a variety of fermentation conditions and then extracting with solvents. Microorganisms have been and still are typically grown in either liquid media (submerged culture) or on solid substrates such as agar or grains. The choice of solvent used for extraction of the secondary metabolites depends on the type of secondary metabolite desired. In order to obtain a broad spectrum of secondary metabolites differing in polarity, a solvent such as methanol can be used for solid fermentations, and butanol can be used for liquid fermentations. Alternatively, resins can be used for extraction of secondary metabolites, with the choice of resin depending on the polarity of the compounds to be extracted. Each natural products group has developed their own fermentation parameters, media, and extraction conditions and as most of this information is not freely available, a general guide is provided below.

3.1.1. Methods for the Preparation of Crude Microbial Extracts

3.1.1.1. FERMENTATION IN LIQUID MEDIA

The microorganism is fermented in liquid media for a certain period of time. To the culture is added an equal volume of butanol and the sample mixed for 30 min to 1 h. The sample is then centrifuged and the solvent (top layer) is removed and dried down under a stream of nitrogen. The sample is then re-suspended in the solvent of choice for the screening deck.

3.1.1.2. GROWTH ON A SOLID SUBSTRATE

The microorganism is grown on a solid substrate such as agar for a certain period of time. To the culture is added a 50% volume of methanol and the sample allowed to stand for 1 h. The liquid is decanted and dried down under a stream of nitrogen. The sample is then re-suspended in the solvent of choice for the screening deck.

3.1.2. Methods for the Preparation of Crude Plant Extracts

The overall procedures for the extraction of plant samples consist of a number of seemingly simple steps. However, careful execution of these steps is critical to ensure that the resulting sample is suitable for HTS *(8)*. In most cases plant material is first dried in the atmosphere, either at room temperature or in an oven at no higher than 30°C. The sample should be not be compacted to avoid fungal infections and elevated temperatures. The sample can be ground or frozen with liquid nitrogen and pounded in a chilled mortar. By reducing the particle size, solvent penetration is more efficient and greater yields of secondary metabolites are achieved. There are many approaches to solvent selection depending on the desired metabolites and these are well-covered elsewhere *(8)*. In general, aqueous-methanol is usually the solvent mixture of choice for the preparation of crude plant extracts. The plant crude extracts at this stage contain tannins, fats, waxes, and chlorophyll and their suitability for use in HTS is debatable.

For both microbial and plant samples, the use of solvents extracting the majority of the secondary metabolites, regardless of their polarity, satisfies the purists who are concerned with losing some of the components as a result of further processing. The disadvantage is that the crude extract is complex and de-convoluting (dereplication) of the hit is a time-consuming process. All natural product groups have their own procedures for dereplicating an activity from a crude extract *(9)*. It is usually necessary to perform bioassay-guided fractionation, which relies on additional resource from screening personnel at a time when the screen may no longer be running, extending the timelines for the program (*see* **Fig. 2**). Dereplication almost always requires some sort of separation step resulting in separation of compounds. This can be done by gravity flow chromatography, fast protein liquid chromatography (FPLC), high-performance liquid chromatography (HPLC), etc. The samples are collected and correlated to regions of the chromatography profile. Once the active region of this profile is determined, the UV/visible spectrum of the peak(s) are compared with a database available either commercially or developed in-house *(10)* to determine if it is a known compound. There are a number of commercial databases that are capable of performing a search based on UV/visible spectrum and molecular weight for the identification of microbial products. These include Bioactive Natural Products Database (Berdy), which lists 23,000 compounds; Antibase™ Database containing 21,000 microbial metabolites; Kitasato Microbial Chemistry Database with 16,000 entries; and the DEREP Database containing 7,000 compounds with a planned expansion to 15,000. Although molecular weight is the most definitive information, the UV/visible absorption data can often result in an exact match. Difficulties can arise when there are nuisance compounds present such as fatty acids, detergents, and pigments. These can cause a false-positive result, usually slow down the isolation process because of their presence in very low amounts, and may be masked with other compounds *(2)*. Historically, it has been through the use of crude

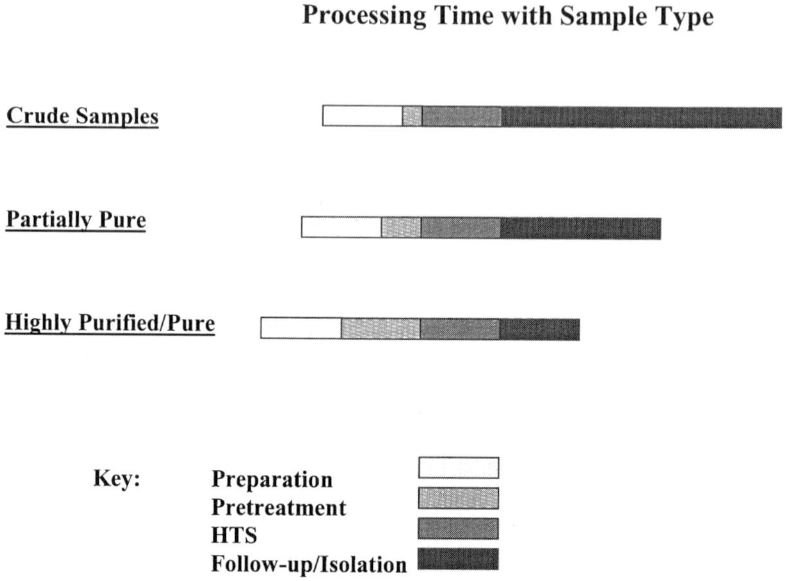

Processing Time with Sample Type

Fig. 2. Schematic showing timelines for screening programs utilizing natural-products samples treated variously prior to entering the screening stream.

extracts as screening samples that the natural products present as drugs in the marketplace today were discovered. However, the screening environment at the time of their discovery was very different from the present screening paradigm, which requires much shorter timelines and the need to know the chemotype at an early stage in the screening process.

3.1.2. Methods for Screening and Evaluating Crude Natural Product Samples

In order to run natural product crudes as samples in screens, a very careful evaluation for tolerance in the screen is required. This entails running 2,000–5,000 samples through the screen at several concentrations to establish the concentration for the HTS. The goal is to run the crude at the highest possible concentration tolerated by the screen; this allows any particular molecule to be run at the highest possible concentration. The dilution series data are treated to generate a normal curve by evaluating how many samples were active at any given level, so, x-axis representing signal and y-axis representing test sample value relative to control. The curve that is the tightest normal distribution will be the concentration to choose. This enables the screener to have a high level of confidence that outlying points are genuine actives and that nonspecific effects are not too interfering.

A **B**

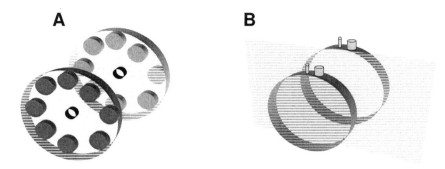

Fig. 3. Schematic of equilibrium microdialysis apparatus. (**A**) Plexiglass rotating cells containing eight walls. (**B**) Schematic of a single well with dialysis film shown between the open halves. One side is loaded with the solvent and natural product, and the other side loaded with vehicle. Entry and exit holes are shown for each half-well and the well are loaded by syringe or sequencing gel-loading tips. These openings are then sealed and the cell is rotated until equilibrium is reached.

Obviously, before committing resources to isolating active principles from crude extracts one might want to eliminate high molecular weight entities. We developed a method that can estimate the molecular weights of the active materials in the milieu of the crude extract, avoiding wasting resource effort on preliminary isolation studies (**Fig. 3**) *(11)*. Using overnight equilibrium microdialysis, and testing both the dialysate and the filtrate samples, one can very easily determine activity on the two sides of a dialysis membrane with a given cutoff. For routine use in evaluating natural product crude samples, either a 1200 or a 3500 MWCO membrane was utilized.

3.2. Partially Purified Extracts: Advantages and Disadvantages

A number of groups prepare partially purified mixtures of microbial secondary metabolites as a means of providing a less complex sample for screening, but not excluding the more minor components. Partially purified mixtures can be obtained by processing the crude extract using either resins or solvents that will separate the components of the mixture based on their polarity *(12)*.

3.2.1. Methods for Preparation of Partially Purified Microbial Extracts

The fermentation is extracted with a polar solvent as described earlier. The butanol extract is then applied to an HP-20 cartridge followed by step gradient dilution, first with 100% water, and then with increasing amounts of methanol, and finally with methanol and acetone to generate essentially water soluble, polar, moderately polar, and nonpolar fractions. These different fractions can be submitted for screening *(10)*. An alternative approach is to use a solvent spartitioning protocol which will also separate components based on their polarity *(12)*. The advantage of these approaches is that the sample is less complex and more concentrated, and therefore there is a greater chance of detecting the relevant biological active entities. The length of time needed for the isolation of the active entity is somewhat reduced, and for the purists there is less chance of overlooking a component from the original mixture than if further manipulation was done.

3.2.2. Methods for the Preparation of Partially Purified Plant Extracts

3.2.2.1. GENERAL PROCEDURE TO OBTAIN A DETANNIFIED CHLOROFORM EXTRACT FROM A PLANT METHANOLIC EXTRACT

The plant is extracted with methanol as described earlier. The resulting aqueous-methanol extract is then defatted with a nonpolar solvent such as hexane or petroleum ether. The hexane layer (containing the fats, waxes, and chlorophylls) is discarded and the aqueous-methanol layer is evaporated and partitioned against chloroform. This results in an aqueous extract that is then washed with 1% aqueous NaCl and dried over anhydrous Na_2SO_4, and a chloroform extract that has been "detannified." Both of these extracts can be submitted for HTS *(8)*.

3.2.2.2. GENERAL PROCEDURE TO OBTAIN A PRECIPITATE OF WATER-SOLUBLE COMPOUNDS SUCH AS SAPONINS FROM PLANTS

The ground plant is directly extracted with chloroform and the extract concentrated to dryness. The gummy residue is then treated with 80% aqueous-methanol, concentrated, and extracted with water-saturated with butanol. To the butanol phase is added ethyl acetate and precipitation of the crude saponins occurs *(8)*.

3.2.2.3. GENERAL PROCEDURE TO OBTAIN ALKALOIDAL EXTRACTS FROM A PLANT METHANOLIC EXTRACT

The methanolic crude extract is treated with 1% aqueous HCl and partitioned against diethyl ether. The diethyl ether phase can be concentrated and contains neutral compounds. The aqueous acid phase is alkalinized with NH_4OH controlling the pH and then partitioned with chloroform. The chloroform extract contains the primary, secondary, and tertiary alkaloids and the aqueous extract contains the quaternary alkaloids, and both of these extracts can be submitted for screening.

3.2.3. Method for Preparation
of Partially Purified Microbial and Plant Extracts

Supercritical Fluid Extraction (SFE) is being used as a general extraction strategy for a wide range of metabolites from plant and microbial samples *(13)*. This approach offers many advantages in that it leads to lower solvent usage, controllable selectivity, cleaner extracts, and less thermal degradation as compared to conventional solvent extraction and steam-distillation methods. The essential components of a typical SFE include a carbon dioxide source, a pump, an extraction vessel, a restrictor, and an analyte-collection vessel, and various SFE systems are commercially available *(13)*. Into the extraction vessel is placed the matrix to be extracted, which could be plant material or fermentation broth. Some preliminary sample preparation may be required, for instance grinding, drying, or even wetting. If the sample is a fermentation broth it must be immobilized onto a solid support, since SFE is generally unsuitable for liquid samples because of difficulties in handling two phases under pressure. The sample is then extracted generally with at least three extraction-cell volumes, in static, dynamic, or re-circulating modes. The extraction cell is usually an oven so that the temperature can be controlled. As the supercritical carbon dioxide passes through the restrictor, the change in pressure in the restrictor causes the pressure of the supercritical fluid to decrease. The analyte is then swept into an on- or off-line collection device. With on-line collection, an analytical instrument such as a gas chromatography (GC), SFC, or HPLC is connected, and the analyte is then analyzed. For the purposes of preparing partially purified mixtures of plant and microbial crude extracts, an off-line collection would be used.

The advantage of using SFE is the removal of deleterious nuisance compounds such as tannins, waxes, and fats from plant material, and fatty acids from microbial fermentations *(13)*. These compounds can give rise to false positive results and mask truly active components, and therefore their removal is of value in the preparation of samples for HTS. The disadvantage is that this procedure is somewhat lengthy and would require some level of automation to be used for numerous samples.

3.3. Relatively Pure Compounds: Advantages and Disadvantages

The logical step in moving away from crude or even partially purified extracts is to produce relatively pure compounds that can be an integral part of the screening deck. There are a number of sources of relatively pure or pure natural products that are commercially available for screening. In addition a number of pharmaceutical companies have developed their own "purified natural product deck," the information about which is proprietary.

One source of pure natural products is the Natural Product Pool *(14)* the creators of which expect to gain major impact in current lead discovery efforts in the pharmaceutical industry in Germany. In this endeavor, the samples are organized in a 96-well microtiter plate format containing 1 mg quantities of each compound together with a database covering the chemical/physical data, biological activities known to date, references, and suppliers. The collection contains natural products as well as carefully selected compounds from chemical synthesis in order to achieve maximum structural diversity. In order to minimize dereplication, special emphasis has been placed on selection of compounds that are biologically active secondary metabolites, although there are new compounds and compounds with patent applications pending. As of June 1997, the Natural Product Pool comprised approx 1700 compounds from microorganisms, plants, marine or aquatic sources, animal sources, natural-product derivatives, and synthetic compounds. The compounds range in molecular masses from 200–400 daltons, and to ensure structural diversity the pool contains representative compounds from most biosynthetic pathways together with classification of the compounds according to chemotype. A number of groups have formed a collaboration to construct this collection of compounds including GBF, Analyticon, and the Universities of Gottingen and Tubingen, among others. The compounds are then commerically available to industrial users, which have included Asta Medica, Boehringer Ingelheim, Boehringer Mannheim, E. Merck, Schering, and AgrEvo.

Another approach to the construction of a natural-product deck of relatively pure or pure compounds is to use novel microbial and plant sources. The microorganisms could be cultured under a variety of conditions based on the experiences of the natural products group. Extracts of both plants and microbes could be prepared in a manner similar to those described earlier. The natural product group at Glaxo Wellcome has moved away from random HTS of uncharacterized extracts, towards smaller targeted sample sets. Prefractionation of these samples takes place prior to screening where appropriate in order to be more compatible with the changes in HTS within the company *(15)*. At Glaxo Wellcome a high-throughput prefractionation program has been implemented that utilizes preparative reverse-phase high-performance (or high pressure) liquid chromatography (RP-HPLC) to fractionate crude extracts. The resulting UV absorbance chromatogram is visually examined and discrete components are selected for inclusion in the sample library, bulking fractions where appropriate. The fractions for submission for HTS include those with sufficient weight and apparent purity by the HPLC/UV *(15)*.

Using preparative HPLC as a means of fractionating the crude extract means that nuisance compounds such as chlorophyll can be eliminated due to their characteristic UV and retention time. In addition for the fractions submitted to the screening deck there are chemical characteristics associated with each fraction that can be used as an aid in either dereplication or as a guide to further isolation work if the biological activity merits.

A commercially available system for separating natural products is the SEPBOX *(16)*. The system was designed with five major specifications: that the total process should provide almost pure compounds in under one day, be completely automated, cover the entire spectrum of compound polarities, provide isolated compounds of sufficient material for structure elucidation, and be able to accommodate all extract types *(16)*. With the SEPBOX, extracts are absorbed on reverse phase materials placed in a pre-column to allow continuous elution based on polarity. The main separation on reverse-phase material of medium polarity produces 18 fractions. Each of these fractions is further fractionated using five to six separation materials. Compounds eluted from these columns are collected into tubes or 96-well plates. Special techniques are required to trap the highly polar fractions. Light-scattering detection is used to characterize the compounds *(16)*.

The advantages of spending time to generate relatively pure or pure natural product compounds in a deck is that the biological data such as potency, IC_{50} values, and specificity is much more meaningful, and allows for comparison with data from synthetic compounds early in the screening process. As shown schematically in **Fig. 2**, the current screening paradigm using pure or nearly pure natural products provides for faster speeds, not only in the initial screening, but also in the subsequent follow up work. With the timelines demanded by a modern HTS program, there is not usually the luxury of having a screen wait for a long period of time while the structure of a natural product is determined, before deciding which of the synthetic or natural product compounds are worth following further. By having the natural-product samples relatively pure, this time can be significantly reduced. Ensuring that the natural products samples are structurally characterized to a degree similar to the other compounds in the deck will enable a larger number of targets to utilize this sample type. In addition, with the move to greater miniaturization of the assay volumes in screens, sample purity will become more of an issue as crude mixtures will not be compatible with the submicroliter volumes that will come from moving from 384-well plates to 1536- and 3456-well plates.

The disadvantages of this approach is that the majority of the purification work is done prior to submission to screening without the guarantee of there being any biological activity. In the past using crude extracts there was detection of biological activity in the sample of interest and this guided the selection of natural product samples to follow. However, with the ever-increasing number of screens that are run each year in the pharmaceutical industry, a deck of sufficient quantities of purified natural products could see hundreds of targets, and therefore warrant the effort. Although using this approach means that fewer organisms and plants end up being included, incorporation of a chemical prescreening step prior to the preparative HPLC stage results in only the most promising extracts being prepared.

3.4. Flow for UHTS

In order to gain an appreciation of the differences the sample type for natural products makes on the timelines in the screening process, the different approaches are compared (**Fig. 2**). It is apparent that for crude extracts from both plants and microorganisms time has to be spent to deconvolute this incredibly complex mixture. At one end of the spectrum, with crude extracts the time is spent after the identification of biological activity, whereas at the other end of the spectrum for relatively pure samples the majority of the work is done prior to the sample being screened. Although there may be a strong need for the natural products group to generate samples that satisfy their needs in terms of how inclusive the sample is, the ultimate destination of that sample, and the environment in which it will be screened has to be kept in mind to ensure that the sample is compatible, and this may require some compromise on the preparation and content of the sample.

4. Examples

Are there unique attributes for natural-products identified as screening hits? Yes.

Special attributes for natural-products identified in HTS programs include: 1) unanticipated and unusual mechanisms of action, 2) the molecular diversity may be synthetically inaccessible, even semisynthetically. Below are examples of (1) and (2). Another clear advantage is the frequent occurrence of analogues, i.e., related compounds found as secondary metabolites in the same culture fermentation.

Examples of (1) are the "activators" of glucokinase, Glucolipsin A and B *(17)*. Glucose phosphorylation influences circulating blood glucose levels, making glucokinase regulation one of the principle points for therapeutic intervention in diabetes. A trivial way to "activate" glucokinase would be to remove a negative allosteric effector from the assay. These two nov el natural products

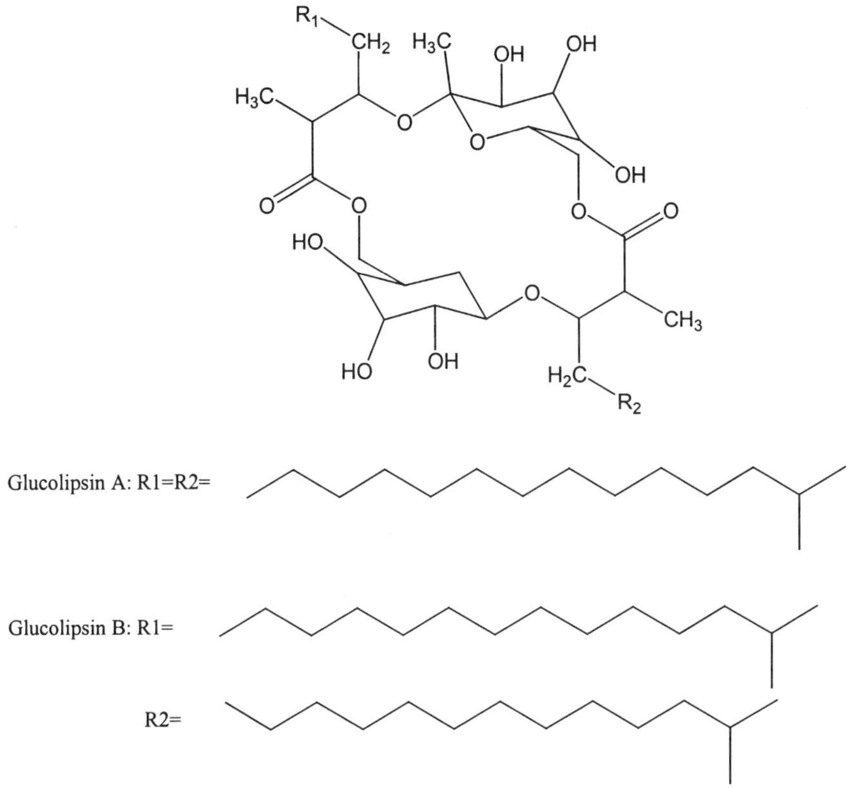

Fig. 4. Structures of two novel natural products that "activate" glucokinase.

exhibit a sequestering activity for one type of negative effector molecules for glucokinase, fatty acyl CoA esters (**Fig. 4**).

A novel member of the ergot alkaloid family, 1-methoxy-5R,10S-agroclavine, was found to be a very selective and potent inhibitor of the Lck tyrosine kinase *(18)*. Inspection of the two-dimensional line drawings for 1-methoxy-5R,10S-agroclavin, and alkaloids such as 5R, 10R-agroclavine, and lysergol, compounds very closely related to LSD or lysergic acid diethlyamide, suggest a structure/activity relationship (**Fig. 5**). Neither 5R,10R-agroclavin or lysergol, which have a trans C/D ring juncture, showed any inhibitory activity toward the Lck tyrosine kinase, nor did they inhibit the autophosphorylation of related kinases. Further studies led to the complete structural elucidation of 1-methoxy-5R,10S-agroclavin. **Figure 6** compares the 3-D structures by line drawing of 1-methoxy-5R,10S-agroclavin and 5R,10R-agroclavin. The drastic three-dimensional structural difference because of the opposite C/D ring junctures may

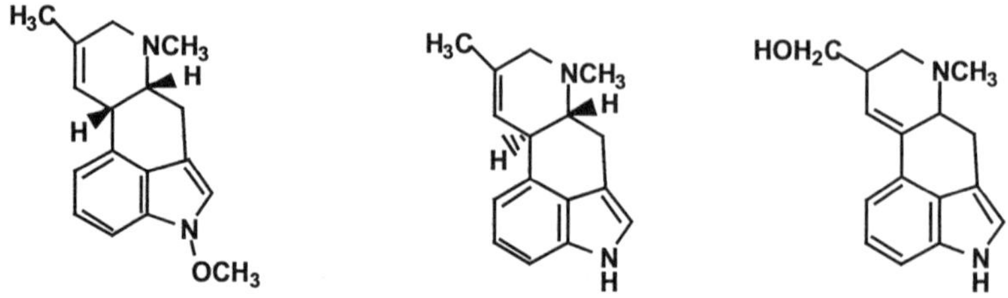

1-methoxy-5R,10S agroclvin   5R,10R agroclavine   lysergol

Fig. 5. Line drawings of 1-methoxy-5R, 10S-agroclavin, and related ergot alkaloids.

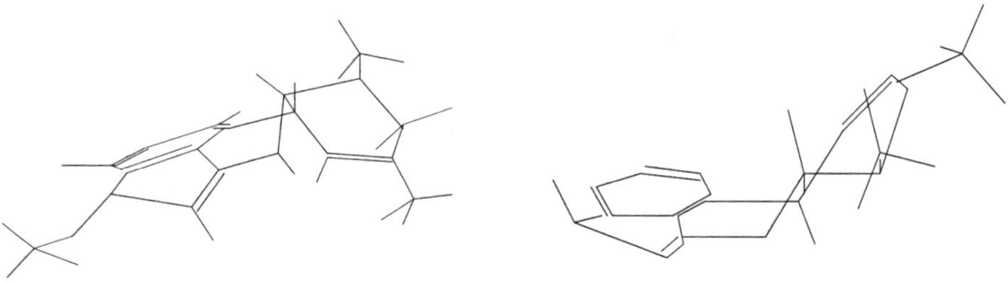

1-methoxy-5R, 10S agroclavin   5R, 10R agroclavin

Fig. 6. Three-dimensional structure of 1-methoxy-5R, 10S-agroclavin, and 5R, 10R-agroclavin.

contribute to the observed enzyme specificities of these compounds. This sort of ring configuration represents a significant challenge synthetically and semi-synthetic methods were not found viable.

5. Conclusions

So, natural products or not? This chapter reviewed methods for incorporating natural products as samples in HTS programs, both historical and current, including the emerging uHTS approaches. A limited discussion of the value of natural products as a source for discovery of unusual and surprising compounds was included.

It is our conviction that the potential for drug discovery from natural product sources has only begun to be utilized. In the long term, the most successful HTS programs will almost certainly be utilizing this source of samples and will undoubtedly feed compounds with interesting and unusual profiles into the pipelines of the pharmaceutical developers.

Acknowledgments

The authors wish to acknowledge the critical review of the manuscript by Salvatore Forenza and Elizabeth Hall. We would also like to thank Salvatore Forenza for **Fig. 1**. Additionally, we would like to acknowledge other members of the BMS Natural Product Research community, including Li-Ping Chang, Lynda S. Cook, Regina D. Ezekiel, Donald R. Gustavson, Robert M. Hugill, Raouf A. Hussain, Kin S. Lam, Grace A. McClure, Robert W. Myllymaki, Edward J. Pack, Christopher J. Poronsky, Jenny Qian-Cutrone, Y.-Z. Shu, Tom Ueki, and Judith A. Veitch.

References

1. Cragg, G. M., Newman, D. J., and Snader, K. M. (1997) Natural products in drug discovery and development. *J. of Natural Products* **60,** 52–60.
2. Shu, Y.-Z. (1998) Review: recent natural products based drug development: a pharmaceutical industry perspective. *J. Natural Products* **61,** 1053–1071.
3. Manly, S. P. (1997) Point/counterpoint: *in vitro* biochemical screening. *J. Biomol. Screening* **2,** 197–199.
4. Cordell, G. A., Farsnworth, N. R., Beecher, C. W. W., Soejarto, D. D., Kinghorn, A. D., Pezzuto, J. M., Wall, et al. (1993) Novel strategies for the discovery of plant-derived anticancer agents, in *Human Medicinal Agents from Plants* (Kinghorn, A. D., and Balandrin, M. F, eds.) American Chemical Society, Washington, DC, Symposium Series 534, pp.191–204.
5. Farnsworth, N. R. (1990) The role of ethnopharmacology in drug development, in *Bioactive Compounds from Plants* (Chadwick, D. J., and Marsh, J., eds.) Wiley, New York, pp. 2–21.
6. Farnsworth, N. R., Loub, W. D., Soejarto, D. D., Cordell, G. A., Quinn, M. L., and Mulholland, K. (1981) Computer services for research on plants for fertility regulation. *Korean J. Pharmacognosy* **12,** 98–109.
7. Loub, W. D., Farnsworth, N. R., Soejarto, D. D., and Quinn, M. L. (1985) NAPRALERT: computer handling of natural product research data. *J. Chemical Information Computer Sci.* **25,** 99–103.
8. Silva, G. L., Lee, I. S., and Kinghorn, A. D. (1998) Special problems with the extraction of plants. in *Methods in Biotechnology*, vol. 4, *Natural Products Isolation* (Cannell, R. J. P., ed), Humana Press, Totowa, New Jersey, pp. 343–363.
9. Carter, G. T. (1998) LC/MS and MS/MS procedures to facilitate dereplication and structure determination of natural products, in *Natural Products Drug Discovery II. New Technologies to Increase Efficiency and Speed* (Sapienza, D. M., and Savage, L. M., eds.) IBC Communications, Southborough, MA, pp. 3–19.
10. Shu, Y. Z., Hussain, R. A., Myllymaki, R. W., and Vyas, D. M. (1998). Rapid and systematic chemical profiling process for accelerating natural product lead discovery, in *Natural Products Drug Discovery II. New Technologies to Increase Efficiency and Speed* (Sapienza, D. M., and Savage, L. M., eds.) IBC Communications, Southborough, MA, pp. 21–49.

11. Padmanabha, R., Cook, L. S., and Manly, S. P. (1996) Use of equilibrium dialysis to estimate the size of active materials in natural product extracts. *J. Biomol. Screening* **13**, 131–133.
12. Baker, D. D. (1998) Optimizing microbial fermentation diversity for natural products discovery, in *Natural Products Drug Discovery II. New Technologies to Increase Efficiency and Speed* (Sapienza, D. M., and Savage, L. M., eds.) IBC Communications, Southborough, MA, pp. 229–247.
13. Venkat, E. and Kothandarama, S. (1998) Supercritical fluid methods, in *Methods in Biotechnology* vol. 4, *Natural Products Isolation* (Cannell, R. J. P., ed.) Humana Press, Totowa, NJ, pp. 91–109.
14. Koch, C., Neumann, T., Thiericke, R., and Grabley, S. (1998) A central natural product pool: new approach in drug discovery strategies, in *Drug Discovery from Nature* (Grabley, S., and Thiericke, R., eds.) Springer-Verlag, Berlin, Heidelberg, pp. 51–55.
15. Stead, P. (1998) Increasing efficiency in natural products lead discovery, in *Natural Products Drug Discovery II. New Technologies to Increase Efficiency and Speed* (Sapienza, D. M., and Savage, L. M., eds.) IBC Communications, Southborough, MA, pp. 51–73.
16. Muller-Kuhrt, L. (1998) Automated isolation as the key approach to make natural product screening more competitive, in *Natural Products Drug Discovery II. New Technologies to Increase Efficiency and Speed* (Sapienza, D. M., and Savage, L. M., eds.) IBC Communications, Southborough, MA, pp. 75–98.
17. Qian-Cutrone, J., Ueki, T., Huang, S., Mookhtiar, K. A., Ezekiel, R. D., Kalinowski, S. S., et al. (1999) Glucolipsin A and B, two new glucokinase activators produced by *Streptomyces Purpurogeniscleroticus* and *Nocardia Vaccinii*. *J. Antibiotics* **523**, 245–255.
18. Padmanabha, R., Shu, Y. Z., Cook, L. S., Veitch, J. A., Donovan, M., Lowe, S. E., et al. (1998) 1-Methoxy-Agroclavine from *Penicillium sp.* WC75209, a novel inhibitor of the Lck tyrosine kinase. *Bioorganic Med. Chem. Lett.* **8**, 569–574.

10

Introduction to Screening Automation

Steven Hamilton

1. History of Screening Automation

In the late 1970s and early 1980s, the components that have made modern high-throughput screening (HTS) laboratory possible came together. Those were: 1) small scale servo-driven robotic devices; 2) the personal computer; and 3) the microplate. The word "robot" is derived from the Czechoslovakian word Robota, which is translated into English as servant, slave, or laborer. The Robot Institute of America (RIA) defines a robot as a "reprogrammable multi-functional manipulator capable of moving materials, parts, or tools through variable programmed motions for the performance of a variety of tasks" *(1)*. The technology for servo-controlled robotics was developed in the late 1960s, and employed in the automotive assembly industry. In the 1970s the development of the microprocessor drastically decreased the cost and scale of the control systems for such robotics, making smaller robots feasible. Cartesian robots had three degrees of freedom (XYZ) and were usually mounted in an XYZ frame. Cylindrical robots had four degrees of freedom: rotation at the base and wrist, elevation, and lateral movement, thus defining a workspace similar to a cylinder. Articulating robots added yet another (fifth) degree of freedom, mimicking the human arm with shoulder, elbow, and wrist rotation. The shoulder joint is mounted on a base allowing the entire arm to rotate. The wrist motion has both pitch and roll, allowing complex movements that were desired at the time by the automotive and electronics industry. The Microbot Alpha was an early small articulated robotic arm intended for educational use that sold for about $5000, and was used in 1981 in the first published example of robotic laboratory automation *(2)*. Zymark Corporation (Hopkinton, MA) created their own cylindrical geometry robotic arm controlled by their proprietary "personal

From: *Methods in Molecular Biology, vol. 190: High Throughput Screening: Methods and Protocols*
Edited by: W. P. Janzen © Humana Press Inc., Totowa, NJ

computer" and began marketing to the laboratory market in 1982 *(3)*. Although the first 96-well plastic plate was created in 1952 at the N.I.P.H in Hungary, it wasn't until 1974 that the format was first used for an enzyme-linked immunoserbent assay (ELISA) assay in London and at the Centers for Disease Control (CDC).

1.1. Natural Products Screening

Some of the earliest pharmaceutical screening automation was developed to search natural-product libraries for active compounds. Most, if not all, of this automation was custom-developed in-house and not published due to the competitive nature of the work Thus no common format or technology arose from these efforts. One published case, by scientists at Eli Lilly and Company (Indianapolis, IN) *(4)*, utilized a PUMA 560 robot to inoculate microbial colonies into vials, leading to a downstream testing of the fermentation extract for antibiotic activity.

1.2. Early Microplate Automation

The first published examples of robotic microplate automation were presented at the Fourth International Symposium on Laboratory Robotics in 1986 *(5–8)*. All were examples of ELISA automation, and while not focused toward compound screening, contained the roots of today's HTS. Using versions of Zymark's early microplate management system, these were examples of how robotic technology was initially used in the laboratory as a "one-armed chemist" *(9)* to anthropomorphically mimic human tasks. Through the use of interchangeable "hands," the robot arm was directly involved in many laboratory unit operations (LUO's) *(1)* such as single and multi-channel pipetting, plate washing, reagent dispensing, and pipet tip attachment/detachment. This approach limited throughput to several tens of plates/d. Reliability for unattended operations was moderate due to the many nonideal operations thrust upon the robotic arm.

1.3. Advent of Microplate-Focused Workstations

It was immediately obvious that the core of microplate automation lay in liquid handling, and equally obvious that articulated robotics arms were not the cost-efficient way to automate this process. Several companies created specialized cartesian-geometry liquid-handling robots. Beckman Instruments (Fullerton, CA) developed the most microplate focused device in the Biomek™ 1000, which offered interchangeable single and multichannel pipetting tools and an integral spectrophotometer. Other companies, such as Hamilton Co. (Reno, NV) and Tecan Inc. (Research Triangle Park, NC) developed more general-purpose devices which initially featured single-channel, fixed-tip liquid handling. Compared to attaching liquid-handling "hands" to articulated robots, these dedicated cartesian geometry systems offered much faster and higher-quality liquid transfer, but a more limited set of LUOs. Thus "workstations" were differentiated as specialized robotic devices focused on a limited set of LUOs vs general purpose robots capable of executing many different LUOs and transporting more than liquids.

The workstation technology immediately found acceptance in early molecular biology/genomics efforts, due to the low-throughput, liquid-handling intensive nature of the work *(10)*.

1.4. Evolution of the Transport/Workstation Integrated System

In an effort to make integrated, multiple-LUO, general-purpose robotic systems more reliable and capable of higher throughput, system designers began off-loading sample manipulation tasks from the robot arm to more and more specialized workstations. An early example similar in concept to current HTS automation was developed by Beckman Instruments combining their Biomek™ 1000 liquid-handling robot with a modified Zymate arm, renamed the Biomek SideLoader™. This system, described by McRorie for screening large numbers of molecules using a receptor-binding assay *(11)*, used the robotic arm only for the transport of microplates and pipet tips to and from the Biomek liquid-handler. Later, plate reader and incubator modules were added. This approach represents the realization that general-purpose robotic arms are best at transporting samples, not performing manipulative LUOs. Automated transport of microplates to/from specialized workstations was key in enabling the assay throughput and reliable unattended operation necessary for the evolution of HTS, and remains the basic model for fully integrated assay systems today with variations in the actual transport device. A side effect of parsing out robotic tasks to workstations was a marked increase in the cost of automated systems, reported to be approx $60,000 for an ELISA system in 1986 *(7)* and that today can range from $200,000 to well over $1,000,000.

2. Screening Automation Today

The explosive growth of HTS has led to a great abundance of automation technology, ranging from simple, small, and affordable liquid-handling workstations to very large factory-style integrated systems, with a continuum of options in between. Below is an attempt to classify the current types of offerings and their functions.

2.1. Simple Workstations

This category includes small liquid handling robots with fixed single- and multichannel pipetting, priced under $50,000 from several manufacturers

(**Appendix 1**). These are directed toward non-HTS operations such as assay development, and are meant to be "personal" workstations with simple software and small footprints. Also included in this category are other single-task devices such as plate washers and reagent dispensers.

2.2. Standard Workstations

Priced approx from $50,000–150,000, these liquid-handling workstations compare to simple workstations by: 1) larger size, still designed to fit on a laboratory bench (up to 1 meter in length, 30" depth); 2) larger work surface; 3) more feature-rich GUI-style software; 4) variable span and individually addressable multichannel pipetting; 5) washable or disposable pipetting tips; and 6) liquid-level sensing. Workstations in this category may have two rather than one robotic pipetting arm. Some include basic ability to move plates about the worksurface, to/from storage devices such as carousels or stackers as well as remove and replace plate lids. Vendors include Tecan, Beckman, Hamilton, and Packard. Also included in this category are 96- and 384-channel liquid handling workstations, which may have most of the features described earlier with the exception of variable-span and individually addressable pipet tips.

2.3. Extended Workstations

These devices are differentiated from standard workstations by: 1) larger size, as long as 2 meters, but still of a depth to rest on a 30" laboratory bench; 2) full ability to move plates to/from devices such as plate readers, washers, hotels, carousels, incubators, and stackers that are built in or attached to the workstation; 3) dual-pipetting arms, one of which may be configured for 96-channel pipetting; 4) software capable of optimally and automatically scheduling the complex interactions of the workstation's feature set; 5) price: from $150,000 to $300,000. These workstations differ from "Integrated Systems" described in **Subheading 2.4.** in that they are limited in their reconfigurability outside of the initially purchased feature set.

2.4. Integrated Systems: Multitasking Robotic Transport

These systems are descendents of the early robotic ELISA approaches, now with the robotic arm acting only to transport microplates and consumables to/from workstations, and are capable of processing tens of thousands of assays per day. These systems are "multitasking" in that one microplate may visit a given workstation multiple times in the course of an assay. This minimizes the number of workstations needed, requires scheduling software to optimize and control the interleaving of processes, and usually causes the robotic transport to be rate-limiting. A great number of liquid-handling workstations, readers, washers, and other devices are today available for integration into these systems, with the limitation primarily the variety of devices a system integrator is able to technically support. As the size and number of workstations in an integrated system has grown to generate increased throughput, robotic arms have been mounted on rails to extend their work envelope. Integrated systems may be as large as 3 meters in length and 2 meters in depth operating on both sides of a rail. Systems of this size require significant open space within a laboratory and usually are built on a specialized, stable table structure. These systems are generally very reconfigurable (with appropriate expertise) and adaptable to new devices due to the flexibility of the robotic arm transport in addressing different device designs. The cost of such systems range from $250,000 upwards.

2.5. Integrated Systems: Linear Transport

An alternative to multitasking integrated system transport is a "linear" transport system. In the full implementation of this model, plates only pass through a given workstation once, and are transported from the starting workstation to the ending workstation in a linear, production-line like manner. This offers maximum throughput, with the rate-limiting step being the slowest workstation operation in the linear chain. For complex assays requiring numerous workstations, the cost of duplicating workstations makes these systems more costly than multitasking systems. However, as assays become less complex, requiring less workstation stages, this price gap narrows or may become nonexistent. The cost of linear-transport devices itself is less than general-purpose robotic arms. Linear systems that operate in this unidirectional manner do not require scheduling software.

Linear transport has been implemented in several ways. The most common is a derivation of true factory-style assembly line transport: a conveyor belt or moving track. The simplicity of conveyor transport systems makes them inherently a more reliable way to move plates among workstations. Workstations must be specifically designed or modified to accept a plate via this mechanism, in some cases with an active mechanism to "lift" the microplate off the track onto the workstation. Thus, these systems tend to be less adaptable to new devices due to the more limited nature of the transport system. Using small robotic arms to move plates to/from devices and the conveyor mechanism increases flexibility but reduces the speed and reliability inherent in a conveyor-based approach. System prices range from around $200,000 for small, focused "mini" systems to several millions of dollars for factory-scale systems.

Another linear approach utilizes multiple small, simple robotic arms to pass plates down the line, from workstation to workstation, not unlike a "bucket brigade." This transport mechanism combines some of the best features of both linear and multitasking systems. The use of a robotic arm at each workstation affords a high degree of flexibility in accessing each workstation, so adaptation to new devices and technology is relatively easy. This approach also allows each workstation/arm unit to be treated as an independent module, which can be combined by the user with one or more other modules to form a variety of workcells based on the task at hand. However this flexibility is not without cost. Placing a capable robotic arm and controlling computer with each module makes this transport technique significantly more expensive than other linear approaches. The current example of this technique is the Zymark Allegro™ system, with prices ranging from $500,000 to over $1,000,000, based on the number of modules purchased.

2.6. Hybrid Approaches

There are several approaches that combine the features of both multitasking and linear transport. The first, currently offered by CRS Robotics Corp. (**Appendix 1**), uses a multitasking robotic arm to move stacks of plates to and from workstations *(12)*. This technique places the workstations, not the robotic arm, in the rate-limiting role, similar to linear systems. Higher throughput can be achieved by simply adding more workstations. A limitation of this approach is that workstations must be capable of accepting and processing stacks of plates.

Linear-transport systems have also been configured to be bidirectional and multitasking to reduce the number of modules required and thereby reducing the cost of the system. In these cases, plates are moved both up and down stream with the linear transport and may re-visit a given workstation multiple times. These systems require scheduling capability just like multitasking robotic-arm transport systems, and differ from robot-based systems primarily in the mechanism of plate movement.

2.7. Detection

Detection is usually the final step of an HTS assay, which may or may not be integrated into an automated system. If an assay produces an end-product that is stable for a defined time, manually moving batches of completed assay plates to a detection device may be a very viable option. Ideally the detection instrument will accept stacks of plates, which is becoming more and more common. This approach simplifies the automated system, which is always desirable, and allows the detection instrument to be used for assays not connected to an automated HTS system.

If the final assay product is not stable, on-line detection is necessary. Most manufacturers of detection instruments today realize that their devices must easily interface with automation, and one can expect the new detection instruments to appear within automated systems fairly soon after introduction. Some detection devices incorporate liquid handling, reagent dispensing, and mixing

LUOs into their feature set, to facilitate very fast timing between final activities and detection. In multitasking systems, the timing of assay steps through detection can be maintained very precisely by the scheduling software. In linear systems, timing will be determined by the rate-limiting workstation, which in some cases may be the detection step.

2.8. Compound Library Storage, Retrieval, and Management

An HTS operation impacts both up and downstream company components. The number of compounds stored in corporate compound collections has grown along with screening capacity. Automation of the storage and processing of these collections becomes necessary to keep up with HTS efforts and minimize tracking and identification errors. The optimal choice of automation will be highly driven by the corporate organizational structure, i.e., whether the compound library and dispersal of samples is centralized or decentralized, whether the screening effort is centralized or decentralized and how geographically distant the various efforts are. In one extreme, the entire compound library may be stored adjacent to a central screening facility, both automated and linked by a plate-transport mechanism. In another extreme, compound storage may be automated only to the extent of bar-coded containers, and compounds are sent out to a variety of screening groups both nearby and around the world.

Technology originally developed for the automated storage and retrieval (ASRS) of industrial parts has been applied to the chemical collections. Some of the earliest examples were in the storage, inventory and processing of plutonium samples *(13)*. Two basic types of ASRS have been employed for large centralized compound libraries. The first example stores multiple compound-containing drawers in a vertical rotary configuration, similar to a ferris wheel. The drawer with the desired compound (along with many others) is rotated to an access door, and extended for either manual or automated retrieval. These units range in height from 6–20 feet, and multiple units can be placed side by side to achieve storage capacity in the millions of compounds. Typically environmental control (humidity, temperature) is achieved by placing these units in an environmentally controlled room (usually custom built). The interface to further downstream automation or manual retrieval may be engineered as a "portal" to maintain environmental control.

The second example of industrial ASRS involves fixed storage racks or shelves, built linearly and to heights of approx 6–20 feet. A retrieval robot with vertical and reach axes of movement travels in front of the racks on a rail, moving samples from the racks to a fixed point at the end of the rail. These are much like automated fork lifts on a rail, having been developed for retrieving large bins or pallets in warehouses. Some models may access racks on both sides of the rail. Environmental control must be achieved for the entire room housing the ASRS. Vendors of these systems include Aurora Biosciences, RTS Thurnall, and REMP.

These large systems, including the facility to house them will typically cost several millions of dollars. In both cases, storage of compounds may be done in bottles, vials, deepwell microplates, or regular microplates, in solid form, or dissolved in dimethyl sulfoxide (DMSO) *(14)*. Solids are usually stored in a sealed vessel at room temperature with controlled humidity. The ideal mode of storing liquid compound libraries is still a topic of much debate, but HTS efforts are driven to work with DMSO-dissolved compounds due the speed of working with liquids vs the laborious nature of solids. Dissolved compounds are usually stored at refrigerated or freezer temperatures, often controlled humidity, and sometimes controlled inert atmosphere. However, below freezing environments and the formation of frost present a challenge for the mechanics of many automated devices. Automated devices for the handling and dissolution of solids do exist (The Automation Partnership), but are not universally applicable to a diverse collection of compounds.

Recently laboratory-scale ASRS devices have been developed. These store 100,000–250,000 compounds in fully automated, environmentally controlled carousels or elevators designed to hold either regular or deepwell microplates. These devices are specifically meant to fit into a normal-size laboratory. Plates are passed to/from the outside world through a portal, which may be integrated to typical plate transport and liquid handling automation. Vendors for these devices include Tecan, Zymark, and TomTec.

Compound library operations are often make large numbers of replicate plates for distribution to screening groups. Automated systems have been developed specifically for this operation, incorporating 96/384-channel pipetting workstations, extensive plate storage, bar-code reading, and applying capability, and plate-sealing technology. These generally fall into the Extended Workstation category described previously, and could be integrated with any of the available ASRS systems.

Any compound inventory system must be linked to a tracking database and often incorporates automated identification (**Subheadings 3.3.** and **3.4.**).

3. Integrating a System

System integration is the art and science of putting together electrical, mechanical, software, and communications technology to create an automated system that addresses the needs of the end-user, is efficient, reliable, and cost-effective. Fully integrated systems, both standard and custom, are available from a variety of commercial sources or one may purchase and/or build components and do the integration oneself if commercial systems are not appropri-

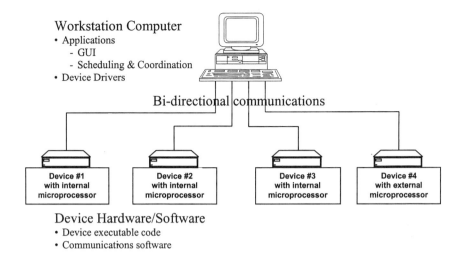

Workstation Computer
- Applications
  - GUI
  - Scheduling & Coordination
- Device Drivers

Bi-directional communications

| Device #1 with internal microprocessor | Device #2 with internal microprocessor | Device #3 with internal microprocessor | Device #4 with external microprocessor |

Device Hardware/Software
- Device executable code
- Communications software

Fig. 1. System software architecture for a workstation. Adapted with permission from *(18)*.

ate. In either case, it is important to understand the fundamentals of system integration either to evaluate commercial systems or to plan and execute your own effort.

3.1. Software and Control

Well-structured automation systems incorporate the concepts of Computer Integrated Manufacturing (CIM) to define workcells and standard protocols to transmit information back and forth between the workcell(s) and the CIM-type software. This model scales to describe systems ranging from Simple Workstations to complex multi-workstation Integrated Systems. **Figure 1** shows this model applied to a workstation, where a central PC is interfaced to a number of devices such as a cartesian robot, syringe pump, peristaltic pump, water bath, and bar-code reader. These devices may have their own imbedded microprocessor and device code or can have this capability added by integrating an analog/digital interface board such as those available through National Instruments. The system PC contains GUI and system management software and drivers for each device. In essence, this is a small "integrated system."

Figure 2 shows this model scaled to a larger system, still controlled by a central computer housing the GUI, scheduling/management software, and device drivers. The only difference in this model is that the PC is interfaced to more complex workstations (i.e., a liquid handler, plate reader, or storage device), transport devices and a network environment. These naturally have more processing power on-board than would a syringe pump in the workstation model.

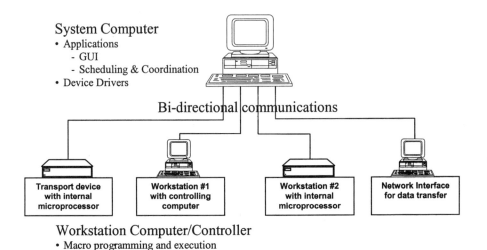

Fig. 2. System Software Architecture for an Integrated. System Adapted with permission from *(18)*.

For example a liquid-handling workstation may have its own controlling PC and programming environment to create macro-level code that can be executed via the drivers on the system PC. But the basic model still remains intact.

The key to this model lies in the separation of the high-level application and driver code (on the system PC) from the lower level hardware, device, or workstation related software or firmware. This creates a modular environment where devices/workstations can be added (or taken out) with software changes only at the higher level, provided that necessary device driver code exists. Early efforts in laboratory automation often found device-related code at multiple levels, making modifications a very difficult and error-prone process.

The high-level system scheduling/management software may be as simple as code to prevent a liquid-handling cannula from colliding with a fixed wash station, or to assure that such a cannula is in liquid to prior to beginning an aspiration step. Such software is not usually apparent to the user. In more complex integrated systems, system scheduling takes on a higher profile and is offered as a specific product. Screening systems conduct multiple operations at several instruments or workstations concurrently, often requiring control over times for reactions, mixing, and incubation. Multitasking systems, i.e., those where the same workstation is used for several stages of the process, require interleaving of samples to maximize system throughput. While it is possible to manually construct such an interleaving schedule, it quickly becomes a difficult Gantt chart exercise for all but simple operations. Software is now available to calculate an efficient interleaved schedule, and translate that schedule into executable code to drive the automated system. This software is nested into the GUI layer of a system and becomes a integral part of setting up and running the automation.

There are several distinguishing features of scheduling software. The most apparent is the style of the GUI. Text-based schedulers allow creation of an operation by choosing from a written list of potential operations or devices by choosing from a list or icon window. The created method "reads" textually like a written laboratory protocol. Graphical or icon-based schedulers offer the creation of an operation via drag and drop of icons or pictures, usually showing some visualization of the device or operation in question. The created method is a flow chart of icons or images, each of which can usually be opened for a verbal description of the operation behind the icon. The choice is a matter of user preference and has no impact on the eventual quality of scheduling. Most scheduling software offers a Gantt chart graphic depicting the completed schedule, estimated run times, either numeric or graphical representations of device percent utilization and postrun information such as error logs and a comparison of scheduled events to actual run-time events.

Scheduling engines can have different features and several levels of sophistication. Following are some of the important distinctions:

1. Linear scheduling: An algorithmic approach that puts the pieces of a schedule together starting with the first step for the first sample, moving step by step forward through the process for all subsequent samples. This is a fairly fast method, but usually does not create the most optimal schedule.

2. Hueristic scheduling: A "forward looking" mathematical approach that considers the entire list of steps and samples as one simultaneous calculation puzzle. Thus an operation at the end of the process, such as an incubation prior to reading can influence the way samples are spaced at the beginning, perhaps leading to a more efficient overall schedule. This calculation approach takes longer and/or more computing power.

3. Hard or variable event times: Some timed events in screening assays must exact, while others allow variance. Good scheduling software allows the user to define the level of variance allowed for each timing step. A window of variability in some steps can aid a heuristic scheduler in finding an optimal solution.

4. Single processes: The ability to schedule only one assay "thread," where only one plate moves from step to next step. Plates may enter or leave the process but multiple plates do not move from step to step. For example, a sample plate is transferred into an assay plate. The sample plate is then discarded or stored and does not continue to the next step while the assay plate continues.

5. Single, parallel processes: The ability to schedule only assay "thread," but allowing the creation of identical parallel tracks within that thread. For example, one sample plate gives rise to two duplicate assay plates, which then follow the same process.

6. Multiple processes: The ability to schedule different processes to run simultaneously or interleaved. For example, one sample plate gives rise to two duplicate assay plates which then follow *different* process.

7. Static schedules: A schedule that is calculated prior to the beginning of the run and whose timing is nonalterable during the course of the run. Because the scheduling is done prior to system operation, time-consuming algorithms can be used to achieve a highly refined schedule.

8. Dynamic schedules: A schedule that is calculated prior to the beginning of the run and whose timing or schedule is alterable or adaptable during the course of the run. The level of adaptability may range from a simple shift of timing due to a minor perturbation (i.e., an automatically recovered error) to complete recalculation of a schedule based on a sensed event (i.e., faster than expected timing, so speed up the schedule) or data input (i.e., based on the data from a plate read, branch to one of several next step options). Definitions of what "dynamic" means vary widely *(16)*. Schedule recalculation on-the-fly must use fast, simpler scheduling algorithms and may therefore produce suboptimal schedules.

9. Simulation features: Many schedulers can execute scheduled code without the system devices actually receiving execution commands. This allows evaluation of the code performance short of actual mechanical movement. Some more sophisticated schedulers will generate a visual computer simulation of the system movement, and may report cases where the executed code would have resulted in a mechanical event such as a crash.

Scheduling software is offered by a number of system integrators (Appendix 1). Most schedulers today are not limited to interfacing with the devices and workstations supported by a specific system integrator. However, integrating one manufacturers scheduler with another's devices requires more in-depth knowledge of the software and driver architecture.

Communication between the system controller and workstations/devices may be accomplished in a variety of ways. The oldest style of interface is an analog signal, often a 4–20 ma current, which can, for instance, be used to control external motor speed. Simple on/off devices such as peristaltic pumps and valves may be controlled using contact closure or TTL (high/low) signals. More complex communications are done using serial, parallel or network pathways. As shown in **Table 1**, serial communications is still the predominant method of device communication, despite being an old technology. This includes RS-232, RS-485 and more recently USB (Universal Serial Bus) and HPSB (High Performance Serial Bus- aka IEEE1394, Firewire). Network connectiv-

Table 1
Percentage of Surveyed Using Different Types
of Electronic Device Communication Modes*[a]*

	1997	1998	1999	Future
Serial	71%	74%	81%	54%
IEEE-488 (parallel)	48	46	53	51
4-20ma (analog)	52	39	37	23
Ethernet	37	38	43	40
USB 7	7	7	15	24
IEE-488HS	–	6	11	11
Other	20	25	38	39

a(Measurement Needs Tracking Survey—Keithley Instruments Inc. 1999)

ity such as Ethernet is growing in popularity, especially for the transmission of large sets of data from plate readers and imagers.

3.2. Error Handling

To take full advantage of the benefits of laboratory automation, unattended operation is often necessary. Such operation, however, requires that more attention be given to error avoidance, detection, correction, and reporting. Choosing a proper strategy must include sound system design, evaluation of sample stability, potential hazards, possibility of instrument damage, and the availability of trained personnel to correct problems *(17)*.

A sound initial design is the best assurance of successful, error-free automation. The fact that additional error-handling capability is the most common system retrofit indicates that system design is often not given enough attention *(18)*. First, equipment appropriate to the task must be chosen. Secondly, the chemical procedure may require modifications to compliment the strengths of the equipment and overcome the weaknesses. Finally, the system must minimize the possibility of automated or human error.

One can expect that errors will occur sometime during the operation of an automated system. The first step toward resolving error situations is detection of the error. Event sensing is one of the basic means of error detection. The appearance or nonappearance of an expected timed event such as data transmission can be a good check of the operation of a system. System schedulers can report and log discrepancies in expected timed events.

Screening systems generally involve moving liquids and objects, such as microplates, and it is desirable to verify that such movement did take place. Switches, optical sensors, and proximity sensors can be used to check operations such as proper valve rotation, the position of incubator doors, and correct placement of a plate prior to extending 96 liquid-handling cannulas into the wells of the plate. Many liquid-handling devices have liquid level-sensing capability, often capacitive, that can assure the cannula is below the air/liquid interface before aspirating. Robotic arms are equipped with some form of tactile feedback, which provides information about the force being exerted by the end-effector driving mechanism. This allows verification of the presence of a microplate or lid in the robotic grippers, and is probably the most widely used method of error detection in a screening system.

When an error is sensed, an appropriate action should be taken. The most desirable response is for the system to correct the problem and continue operation. Programming for error recovery must be sophisticated enough to account for variations in specific failures, including the possibility that the sensed failure is false. For instance, if failure to attach a pipet tip was sensed, an error-recovery routine must first execute a "discard tip" sequence before attempting once again to pick up a tip. Error-recovery routines should be programmed not lead to "error cascades," creating a larger problem than was initially present.

In some cases, automated error recovery may not be desirable, such as when precious compounds or reagents are involved. When an irrecoverable error is encountered, or recovery has been attempted and failed, the system may either bypass the error if this situation has been pre-determined to be acceptable or the system must be halted and the error condition annunciated in some way. Audible and visual alarms are effective where humans are likely to be nearby. Fully unattended systems can be programmed to send error notification through network or telephone connections to pagers, cell phones or e-mail. Systems may be switched back and forth between local and remote annunciation at different times of the day *(19)*.

3.3. Automatic ID

Automated identification is essential in a modern high throughput laboratory. Bar coding has gained wide acceptance in screening labs as a specialized form of sample tracking and error avoidance. Bar coding is a visual representation of a digital code in which bars and intervening spaces represent ASCII (American Standard Code for Information Exchange) characters and symbols. Data transcription using bar codes has been estimated to be 1 billion times more reliable than manually entered data *(20)*.

An identification strategy should be developed before any hardware is purchased. The fundamental choice is whether to use the bar code simply as a "pointer" to information in a database (also known as the "license plate" approach) or to imbed actual information into the bar code. The former strategy has positives such as simplicity and long-term scalability of scheme and the ability to use

Fig. 3. General barcode structure. Adapted with permission from *(18)*.

pre-printed labels of high quality, avoiding the cost of multiple in-house printing devices. Negatives of this strategy include reliance on regular and timely interaction with a database to transact ID data, and little or no human-interpretable information. The latter (imbedded information) strategy requires print-on-demand capability, often at multiple locations. Database interaction is less frequent, but still required to log or execute the creation of a new ID number. The most positive aspect of this strategy is that visual information on the label can identify the plate content without requiring database interaction. The largest downside of this strategy is the potential creation of an ID scheme that "evolves" over time with a tendency to imbed too much information into the label, thus becoming unscalable and unwieldy.

Bar codes are used in laboratories in two different popular formats. Code 3 of 9 (code 39) can express the full alphanumeric character set plus seven special characters (a total of 39). This code is among the least space-efficient and is therefore not always ideal for use on small labels such as microplates. Code 128 can express the full 128 character ASCII set, but more importantly is one of the least space-consuming codes, making it ideal for screening applications. Those considering new laboratory applications should evaluate Code 128 first *(21)*. Both of these code types fit the general bar code structure illustrated in **Fig. 3**.

The demand for more detailed information in bar codes has led to the development of two-dimensional (2D) coding, often called dot or matrix codes. While not yet in the laboratory mainstream, they do represent the direction being taken in some industries, such as the Japanese Medical Association *(22)*. Advantages of 2D code include much higher density of information and a high level of redundancy, which allows a significant portion of the label to be damaged yet still provide complete data. One version of 2D symbology is a stacked

500 characters, 10 mil linear—Code 39

500 characters,
10 mil stacked linear—PDF 417

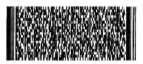

500 characters,
10 mil 2D matrix—Data Matrix ECC 200

Fig. 4. Comparison of Bar Code Symbologies. Adapted with permission from *(26)*.

bar code. These include the first 2D bar code, Code 49, introduced by Intermec Corporation in 1987. Since then additional formats have appeared, including PDF 417 and Code 1. Checkerboard or matrix symbologies can encode as many as several thousand characters in a small amount of space. This code consists of two black bars that intersect at right angles to define the perimeter of the code. Within this boundary, a series of black-and-white squares are written, as illustrated in **Fig. 4**.

Barcode readers are devices that will interpret the bar-code symbol and communicate the interpreted information to the laboratory automation system. The simplest of these devices use a laser or light-emitting diode to illuminate the code and use a light sensitive diode to receive the reflected pulses of light. These readers cannot decode a label that is smudged, torn, or incorrectly applied. More complex imaging devices, such as charged coupled device (CCD) cameras, can read the bar code in any orientation. These cameras have in the past been too expensive for routine use in automated systems, but dramatic price reductions now make them a more practical solution. Imaging scanners are required for many of the 2D code formats, such as Matrix.

The effectiveness of any bar coding strategy can by highly affected by the choice of label stock and the type of printer used. Label stock must be chosen after considering environmental conditions such as temperature, humidity, and chemical exposure. Synthetic stock rather than paper is more durable for a laboratory environment. If the label is to be placed in a freezer environment, the adhesive must remain viable at those temperatures, and also withstand freeze/thaw cycles. The adhesive must also be resistant to flowing around the edges of the label, which can cause errors in automated microplate de-lidding and transport.

Externally printed labels, made by professional printing organizations, offer the highest quality of print resolution and durability. However, this requires an identification strategy that is compatible with pre-printed labels. In-house printing offers a much higher degree of flexibility. Numerous print technologies are available, including dot matrix, direct thermal, thermal transfer, ink jet, and laser printing. Dot-matrix printing will not offer adequate resolution to label most microplates. Direct thermal printing should be avoided since the paper is heat-sensitive. Thermal-transfer printing may be suitable in some cases, but does require a specialized printer as well as costly media and ribbons. A high-quality, single-pass, ribbon-type printer should be chosen to assure highest resolution printing. Laser printers will cost more than thermal transfer printers but do offer very high print resolution and low-cost consumables.

3.4. Data Transport and Management

Data is the ultimate "product" of screening groups, and automation has logarithmically increased the amounts of data being produced. It has also become more common for automated systems to require importation of key operational information. Therefore internal data management and bi-directional data-transfer capability are key features of screening automation (**Fig. 2**). The types of data handled by these systems include inventory, tracking, assay protocols, and measured data. Most commercial automation systems do not include a formal data-management package, but increasingly do provide tools to import and export data using industry standard protocols, such as ODBC compliant files, Excel format, and ASCII flat files. Similarly, most commercial screening data management systems do not offer plug-in data-management integrated with automated systems due to the complexity, specialization, and diversity of automation. This leaves a gap between the laboratory equipment and the database that must be filled by custom programming, often on a case-by-case basis, through either internal or contract resources (23). Some screening groups postpone dealing with this data-interface issue by using easily accessible software packages such as Excel. Inevitably these solutions lead to a crisis as increasingly large and complex data management requirements exceed the feature set of the "easy" tool. It is important to begin planning and executing a long-term data management and automation interface architecture long before the crush of data exists. A number of quality consulting groups have formed to fill the automation-data interface gap. These include Taratec Development Corporation (Bridgewater, NJ 08807); EMAX Solution Partners (Newtown Square, PA 19073); and Integrated Systems Consulting Group (ISCG) (Wayne, PA 19087).

3.5. Facilities

Anyone who has been involved in creating and growing a screening program has found that fully integrated screening systems are not made to fit into a typical wet chemical laboratory. Nor do most laboratories have the full range of services required by many of these systems. The ideal screening laboratory will have:

1. Access to utilities
   a. Compressed air (30 psi, 80 psi)
   b. Water (DI, chilled, heated)
   c. Vacuum (house, local)
   d. Gases
   e. HVAC (special ventilation)
   f. Power (conditioning, surge protection, UPS)
   g. Network
   h. Telephone (modem, pager, remote video)
2. Proper entry and exit for moving equipment
3. Space to walk completely around system
4. Compatibility with people, operation, and safety
   a. Isolate people from equipment
   b. Isolate equipment from people
   c. Isolate people from chemical/biological hazards
   d. Isolate equipment from hazards
      (Chemical, biological, radiological contamination, chemical spills, vapors)
   e. Provide for hazards detection
5. Storage space for disposables, waste and samples
6. Space for component test and repair
7. Preparation workspace

4. Future Direction

Current laboratory automation technology is poised to take the discipline forward for a number of years. The microplate format is almost universal, and all data indicates a deliberate movement toward higher-density microplates. The current transport technology is immediately compatible with higher-density formats, and liquid handling technology is progressing toward routine submicroliter capability. Systems built to handle 96-well microplates do not look greatly different from those designed for 384- or 1536-well microplates. It remains to be seen where practical limitations of hardware and biochemistry constrain the march toward microwell or micro-array approaches, but it is safe to say that microplates and automation to support that assay format will be around for some time to come.

4.1. Microfluidics

An emerging technology that has little lineage with current automation technology is microfluidics. Ironically, microfluidics has much in common with an older chemistry automation technology, flow injection, and segmented flow technology. The migration to nanoliter scale has been made possible largely through advances in micromachining driven by the semiconductor industry. Microfluidic systems are closed pumping systems, thereby having no evaporation problems, unlike microwell approaches. Detection must be sensitive and fast, but has the simpler imaging challenge of a serial sample flow rather than array imaging. The devices are or will be relatively simple, so the addition of parallel channels is not expected to be cost-prohibitive.

Significant challenges do still exist. The liquid handling interface of the macro world to the micro world is far from optimized, and currently tends to waste more sample and reagent than is actually used for the assay. Surface and fluid interactions have a significant effect since the very small flow channels (20–50 micron diameters) create a large surface-to-liquid ratio. One consequence is very strong laminar flow, which makes mixing of liquids difficult. Thermal effects, from the outside world or internally from chemical reactions have a large impact in the nanoworld. Pumping techniques, such as electroosmotic flow, can impact chemical reactions and mixing. The result is that many biochemical reactions behave differently in a microfluidic environment than in a microplate well. Screeners have spent years learning to understand and interpret biochemical and cell-based assay behavior in microplates. The same learning process will have to occur for the microfluidics environment. Early results indicate that the migration is possible, at least for certain classes of assays (*24–25*).

References

1. Hurst, W. J. and Mortimer, J. W. (1987) *Laboratory Robotics: A guide to Planning, Programming and Applications.* VCH Publishers, New York, NY.
2. Owens, G. D. and Eckstein, R. J. (1982) Robotic sample preparation. *Anal. Chem.* **54**, 2347–2351.
3. Hawk, G. L, Little, J. N. and Zenie, F. H. (1982) A Robotic Approach to Automated Sample Preparation. *Am. Lab.* **14,** 96–104.
4. Godfrey, O., Raas, A. and Landis, P. (1987) The application of a robotic work station to the handling of microbial colonies, in *Advances in Laboratory Automation Robotics,* vol. 4 (Strimatis, J. and Hawk, G. L., eds.), Zymark, Hopkinton, MA., pp. 161–174.
5. Hamilton, S. D. (1986) Robotic assays for fermentation products, in *Advances in Laboratory Automation Robotics,* vol. 3 (Strimatis, J. and Hawk, G. L., eds.), Zymark, Hopkinton, MA. pp. 1–23.

6. Hahn, G. D. and Lightbody, B. G. (1986) Automated EIA microplate management system applications of a monoclonal antibody development laboratory, in *Advances in Laboratory Automation Robotics,* vol. 3 (Strimatis, J. and Hawk G. L., eds.), Zymark, Hopkinton, MA, pp. 167–180.

7. Eckstein, R. J., Owens, G. D., Coggeshall, C. W., Macke, B. A. and Miller, K. S. (1986) Making a "turn-key" ELISA robot work, in *Advances in Laboratory Automation Robotics,* vol. 3 (Strimatis, J. and Hawk G. L., eds.), Zymark, Hopkinton, MA, pp. 181–200.

8. Bente, P., Shuman, M., and Schliefer, A. (1986) A robotic microassay system: enzyme linked immunosorbent assays in a 96-well plate format, in *Advances in Laboratory Automation Robotics,* vol. 3 (Strimatis, J. and Hawk, G. L., eds.), Zymark, Hopkinton, MA, pp. 201–216.

9. Freifeld, K. and Kindel, S. (1985) The one-armed chemist. *Forbes* **135,** 116.

10. Shigeura, J. (1989) Mechanical design of small-volume fluid-handling robots for the molecular biology laboratory, in *Advances in Laboratory Automation Robotics,* vol. 6 (Strimatis, J. and Hawk, G.L., eds.), Zymark, Hopkinton, MA, pp. 39–74.

11. McRorie, D. K. and Baudry, M. (1989) Automation of binding assays for glutamate receptor subtypes using the Biomek 1000 laboratory workstation equipped with the Biomek SL robotic arm, in *Advances in Laboratory Automation Robotics,* vol. 6 (Strimatis, J. and Hawk, G.L., eds.), Zymark, Hopkinton, MA., pp. 357–368.

12. Reichman, M., Marples, E., and Lenz, S. (1996) Approaches to automation for high-throughput screening. *Lab. Robotics Automation* **8,** 267–276.

13. Grundmann, J. (1989) Reliability, availabilty and maintainability for a laboratory automated storage and retrieval system. *Lab. Robotics Automation* **1,** 95–104.

14. Janzen, W. (1996) High throughput screening as a discovery tool in the pharmaceutical industry. *Lab. Robotics Automation* **8,** 261–266.

15. Murray, C. and Anderson, C. (1996) Scheduling software for high-throughput screening. *Lab. Robotics Automation* **8,** 295–306.

16. Feiglin, M., Skwish, S., Laab, M., and Heppel, A. (2000) Implementing multilevel dynamic scheduling for a highly flexible 5-rail high throughput screening system. *J. Biomol. Screening* **5,** 39–47.

17. Hamilton, S. D. (1989) Avoiding and handling errors during unattended operation of automated laboratory equipment. *Lab. Robotics Automation* **1,** 53–62.

18. Hamilton, S. D., Kramer, G. W., and Russo, M. F. (2000) *Introduction to Laboratory Automation,* a short course presented at Laboratory Automation 2000, Palm Springs, CA.

19. Hamilton, S. D. (1986) An integrated robotic sample preparation and HPLC analysis of biosynthetic human insulin, in *Advances in Laboratory Automation Robotics,* vol. 4 (Strimatis, J. and Hawk, G. L., eds.), Zymark, Hopkinton, MA, pp. 195–216.

20. Maffertone, M. A., Watt, S. W., and Whisler, K. E. (1990) Automated specimen handling: bar codes and robotics. *Lab. Med.* **21,** 436–443.

21. Collins, D. J. and Whipple, N. N. (1994) *Using Bar Code.* Data Capture Institute, Duxbury, MA.
22. Cost, J. G. (ed.) (1996) *Handbook of Clinical Automation, Robotics and Optimization.* John Wiley & Sons, Inc., New York, NY, pp. 257.
23. Allee, C. (1996) Data management for automated drug discovery laboratories. *Lab. Robotics Automation* **8**, 307–310.
24. Cronin, C. T. (2000) Plastic microfluidic systems for high-throughput genomic analysis and drug screening. Presented at smallTalk 2000, San Diego, CA.
25. Rasnow, B., Li, C., Mayeda, C., Grandsard, P., Pacifici, R., Tagari, P., et al. Screening in LabChips®: early results from the Amgen-Caliper partnership. Presented at smallTalk 2000, San Diego, CA.
26. Scharf, B., Allen, M., and Kenan, P. (2000) Bar Code Technology.

Appendix 1: Technology Providers

North America

Abacus
105 Morse Road
Bennington, VT 05201
Tel: 802-442-3662
Fax: 802-442-8759

Acuity Imaging Inc.
9 Townsend West
Nashua, New Hampshire
Tel: 603-598-8400
Fax: 603-577-5964

Aurora Biosciences Corp.
11010 Torreyana Road
San Diego, CA 92121
Tel: 858-404-6600
Fax: 858-404-6714
www.aurorabio.com

MDS Autolab Systems
100 International Blvd.
Etobicoke, Ontario, Canada
M9W 6J6
Tel: 416-675-4530
Fax: 416-675-0688
www.autolabsystems.com

BioDot Inc.
BioDot, Inc.
17781 Sky Park Circle
Irvine, CA 92614
Tel: 949-440-3685
Fax: 949-440-3694
www.biodot.com

BioRobotics Inc.
12 Walnut Hill Park
Woburn, MA 01801
Tel: 781-376 9791
Fax:781-376 9792
www.biorobotics.com

Bohdan Automation
562 Bunker Court,
Vernon Hills, IL 60061-1831
Tel: 847-680-3939;
Fax: 847-680-1199
www.bohdan.com

Caliper Technologies Corp.
605 Fairchild Drive
Mountain View, CA 94043-2234
Tel: 650-623-0700
Fax: 650-623-0500
www.calipertech.com

Cartesian Technologies, Inc.
17781 Sky Park Circle
Irvine, CA 92614
Tel: 949-440-3680
Fax: 949-440-3694
www.cartesiantech.com

CCS-Packard
24030 Frampton Ave.
Harbor City, CA 90710
Tel: 905-332-2000
Fax: 905-332-1114
www.ccspackard.com

CRS Robotics Corp.
5344 John Lucas Drive
Burlington, Ontario
Canada L&L6A6
Tel: 905-332-2000
Fax: 905-332-1114
www.crsrobotics.com

Cyberlab, Inc.
36 Del Mar Drive
Brookfield, Ct. 06804
Tel: 203-740-3565
Fax: 203-740-3566

CyBio, Inc.
500 West Cummings Park, Suite 1200
Woburn, MA 01801 USA
Tel: 781-376-9899
Fax: 781-376-9897
www.cybio-ag.com
www.cyber-lab.com

EMAX Solution Partners
18 Campus Blvd., Newtown Square
Pennsylvania, 19073
Tel: 610-325-3700
Fax: 610-325-3782
www.emax.com

Hudson Control Group
44 Commerce Street
Springfield, NJ 07081
Tel: 201-376-7400
Fax: 201-376-8265
www.hudsoncontrol.com

Intelligent Automation, Inc.
149 Sidney Street
Cambridge, MA 02139
Tel: 617-354-3830 (ext. 401)
Fax: 617-547-9727
www.automationonline.com

Orchid Biocomputer Inc.
303 College Road East
Princeton, NJ 08540
Tel: 609-750-2200
Fax: 609-750-2250
www.orchidbio.com

Motoman, Inc.
805 Liberty Lane
West Carrollton, Ohio 45449
Tel: 937-847-3300
www.motoman.com

Oyster Bay Pumpworks
One Bay Avenue
P.O. Box 96
Oyster Bay, NY 117711
Tel: 516-922-3789
Fax: 516-624-9253
www.obpw.com

Rixan Associates
7560 Paragon Road
Dayton, OH 45459
Tel: 937-438-3005
Fax: 937-438-0130
www.rixan.com

Beckman Coulter, Inc.
4300 N. Harbor Boulevard
P.O. Box 3100
Fullerton, CA USA 92834-3100
Phone: 714-871-4848
Fax: 714-773-8283
www.beckman.com

Source for Automation
327 Fiske Street
Holliston, MA 01746
Tel: 508-429-3377
Fax: 508-429-5450
www.sourceforautomation.com

Tecan U.S.
P.O. Box 13953
Research Triangle Park, NC 27709
Tel: 919-361-5200
Fax: 919-361-5201
www.tecan-us.com

TekCel
116 South Street,
Hopkinton, MA 01748
Tel: 508-544-7000
Fax: 508-544-2852
www.tekcel.com

TomTec
1010 Sherman Ave.
Hamden, CT 06514
Tel: 203-281-6970
Fax: 203-248 5724

Zymark
Zymark Center
Hopkinton, MA 19350
Tel: 508-435-9500
Fax: 508-435-9761
www.zymark.com

Zymark Ltd.
530 Otto Rd., Unit 8
Mississauga, Ontario L5T 2L5
Canada
Tel: 905-564-1615
Fax: 905-564-1623

Europe

AEA Technology plc
Central House
14 Upper Woburn Place
London, UK
WC1H 0JN
Tel: +44 (0)207 554 5500
Fax: +44 (0)207 554 5570
www.aeat.co.uk

The Automation Partnership Ltd.
Melbourn Science Park
Melbourn, Royston
Hetfordshire SG8 6HB UK
Tel: 44 1763 262026
Fax: 44 1763 262613
www.autoprt.co.uk

Biorobotics Ltd.
Bennell Court
Comberton, Cambridge
CB3 7DS UK
Tel: +44 1223 264345
Fax:+44 1223 263933
www.biorobotics.com

Discovery Technologies Ltd.
Innovation Center, Gewerbestrasse 16
CH-4123 Allschwil
Switzerland
Tel: +41 61 487 8585
Fax: +41 61 487 8599
www.discovery-tech.com

GeSiM mbH, Rossendorder
Bautzner Landstrasse 45
D-01454 Grosserkmannsdorf
Germany
Tel: +49 351 2695 322
Fax: +49 351 2695 320
www.gesim.de

Genetix Ltd.
63-69 Somerford Road
Christchurch, Dorset
BH21 1QU, United Kingdom
Tel: +44 (0) 1202 483900
Fax: +44 (0) 1202 480289
www.genetix.co.uk

ID Business Solutions Ltd.
The Surrey Research Park
5 Huxley Road
GU2 5RE Guildford, Surrey
UK
Tel: +44 1483 595000
Fax: +44 1483 595001

CyBio AG
Goschwitzer Str. 40
D-07745 Jena, Germany
Tel: +49 (0) 3641 65-1400
Fax: +49 (0) 3641 65-1409
www.jenoptik.de

Labman Automation Ltd.
1 Wainstones Court
Stokesley, North Yorkshire TS9 5JY
UK
Tel: +44 1642 710580
Fax: +44 1642 710667
www.labman-automation.com

Matrix Technologies Corp.
13 Croft Road
UK, Wilmslow, Cheshire
SK9 6JJ
United Kingdom
Tel: +44 161 4298162
Fax: +44 161 4770446
www.matrix.com

Process Analysis & Automation Ltd.
Flacon House
Fernhill Road
Farnborough, Hampshire
GU14 9 RX, United Kingdom
Tel: 0252 373000
Fax: 0252 371922

ROBOCON
Labor-und Industrieroboter-Ges.m.b.H.
Davidgasse 85-89
A-1100 Vienna
Austria
Tel: +43 1 641 85 00
Fax: +43 1 641 46 55
www.robocon.com

REMP AG
Burgdorfstr 44
CH-3672 Oberdiessbach
Switzerland
Tel: +41 31 7707070
Fax: +41 31 7712266
www.remp-ch.com

Rosys Anthos
Feldbachstrasse CH-8634
Hombrechtikon, Switzerland
Tel: +41 55 254 2223

Scitec SA
Av. De Provence 20
CH-1000 Lausanne 20
Switzerland
Tel: 41 21 624 1533
Fax: 41 21 624 1549

TECAN AG
Feldbachstrasse 80
8634 Hombrechtikon
Switzerland
Tel: +41 (0)55 254 81 11
Fax: +41 (0) 55 244 38 83
www.tecan.com

Zymark GmbH
Black & Decker Str. 17
65510 Idstein/Ts., Germany
Tel: 011 49 6126 94520
Fax: 011 49 6126 54351

Zymark Ltd.
The Genesis Centre, Science Park
South Birchwood, Warrington, Cheshire,
WA3 7BH, United Kingdom
Tel: 01925-826600
Fax: 01925-826292

Zymark SA
ZAC de Paris-Nord II
13 rue de la Perdrix
B.P. 40016, 95911 Roissy-Charles
de-Gaulle Cedex, France
Tel: 1 48 63 71 35
Fax: 1 48 63 71 53

Asia

Nissel Sangyo Co. Ltd.
24-14 Nishi-Shimbashi 1-Chome
Minato-Ku, Tokyo, Japan
Tel: (03) 3504-7261
Fax: (03) 3504-7745

Integrated Sciences Pty Ltd
2 McCabe Place
Willoughby, NSW 2068, Australia
Tel: 02-9417 7866
Fax: 02 9417 5066
www.integratedsci.com.au

BM Equipment
25-4 Hongo 3-chome
Bunkyo-ku, Tokyo, Japan 113-0033
Tel: +81-3-3818-5091
Fax: +81-3-3818-5530

Kyong Shin Scientific
302 Kyon Shin Bldg, 982-1
Shinwol 7-dong, Yangchun-gu,
Seoul, Korea
Tel: +82 2 608 5868
Fax: +82 2 695 1646

Genasia Scientifics Inc
F3, 166 Chern Kong Road
Sec 3, Nei-Hu
Taipei, Taiwan
Tel: +886 2 2795 1330
Fax: +886 2 2795 276

11

Unit Automation in High Throughput Screening

Karl C. Menke

1. Introduction

This chapter will explain the unit automation approach to high throughput screening. The unit automation approach is predicated on the belief that automation is best implemented only to the extent that operations are standardized, i.e., if you standardize individual assay steps (or unit operations) they can be readily (and effectively) automated (*1*). If entire assay formats could be standardized, then it would make sense to automate the entire assay. However, unless assay development is severely constrained this is not possible. We have found that the majority of scientists will not agree on a standardized protocol for a particular assay format, therefore we have chosen to automate only to the level of unit operations. It should be noted that the concept of identifying, standardizing, and optimizing unit operations is applicable to fully automated screening systems as well.

2. Unit Automation Defined

2.1. Automating the Process Rather than the Assay

Unit automation can perhaps best be described by contrasting it with the alternative methodology of integrated automation. In integrated automation, samples, reagents, plates, and other consumables are supplied to an integrated system of liquid-handling instruments, detectors, and robotic plate manipulators (*2*). Scheduling software then controls the flow of plates through the system and conducts the entire assay, totally unattended in the best of cases. Several different assay protocols may be conducted in parallel. Human intervention is limited to feeding test samples, plates, and reagents and disposing of waste.

From: *Methods in Molecular Biology, vol. 190: High Throughput Screening: Methods and Protocols*
Edited by: W. P. Janzen © Humana Press Inc., Totowa, NJ

In contrast, the unit automation approach is limited to automating individual workstations that perform a single unit operation. In unit automation, each workstation is an island of automation that is designed to optimally perform a single function for maximal throughput *(3)*.

2.2. Plate Handling is the Biggest Difference

The single biggest difference between unit automation and fully integrated automation is in the approach to plate handling. In unit automation, the individual workstations have dedicated plate-handling capability to move a number of plates through that particular unit operation. The plate-handling may be performed by stackers, conveyers, robotic manipulators, and carousels, or other means. The difference is that human beings are used to move the batches of plates from one unit operation to the next.

2.3. Standardization of Equipment and Methods is Key

As mentioned earlier, the key to effective implementation of automation is standardization. Standardization of both equipment and methods used is a great enabler of further improvements in effectiveness.

Standardizing on the equipment to be used for a given unit operation has many advantages and benefits.

- Identify standards for future purchases
- Identify equipment types that need investigation
- Prioritize integration and development of tools
- Reduce complexity and proliferation of required support skills
- Consolidate sourcing and service
- Toolbox for screen development
- Process for evaluating new equipment

Method standardization is as simple as picking one methodology and sticking to it wherever possible. Once a standard method has been identified, it can be optimized, tweaked, and refined. By reusing a standard methodology, progression up the learning curve is cumulative, rather than starting anew with each new assay. Departure from the standard method should only be permitted when there is a valid reason for the exception. For example, there is minimal benefit and great complexity if custom plate maps are developed for each assay to be run in dose-response mode.

3. What are Unit Operations?

Unit operations are those individual process steps that make up an assay protocol. Unit operations can be standardized in terms of both equipment uti-

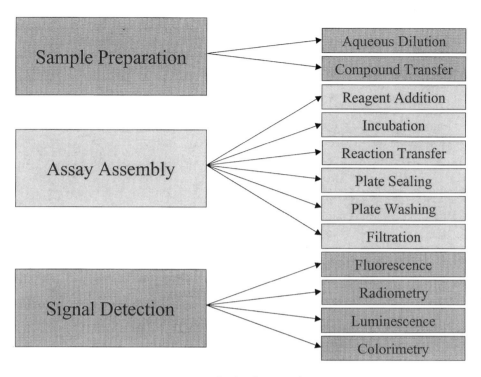

Fig. 1. Typical unit operations.

lized and methodology. Typically, unit operations in HTS can be divided into three categories: 1) sample preparation, 2) assay assembly, and 3) signal detection (*see* **Fig. 1**) *(4)* Very simple homogenous assay formats (sometimes referred to as mix-and-measure) may just involve additions, incubation, and reading. More complex heterogeneous formats may include many more steps involving filtration, plate-washing, plate-to-plate transfers, etc. The point is that unit operations are the building blocks that can be combined in whatever order is needed for a particular assay protocol. Once unit operations are defined and standardized, they can be effectively automated with little or no dependence on the particulars of a given assay.

Process flowcharting can be used to graphically represent an overview of an assay protocol. The format shown in **Fig. 2** uses the convention of materials flowing in from the left, waste streams exiting to the right. Additionally, information on critical parameters, equipment used, and throughput for each unit operation is represented.

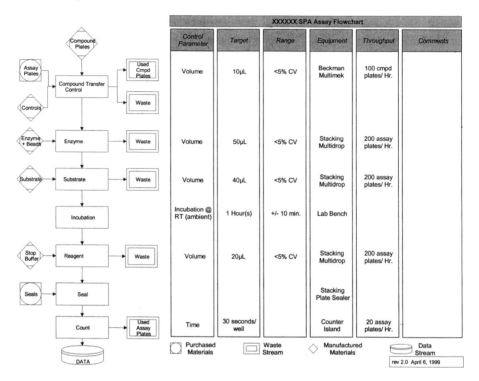

Fig. 2. Assay process flowchart.

3.1. Sample Preparation

Sample preparation unit operations include those steps necessary to provide the test samples in the proper volume, concentration, and diluent for screening. Examples include:

- Transferring aliquots of sample (generally in 100% dimethyl sulfoxide [DMSO]) from compound library stock plates to a sample plate.
- Diluting the sample plates with aqueous buffer.
- Serial dilution of test samples (for multipoint dose-response curves).
- Transferring aliquots of the diluted sample and assay controls to the assay plate.

3.2. Assay Assembly

Assay assembly unit operations include all the steps necessary to combine the test samples with all the other ingredients of the assay. Examples of assay assembly unit operations include the following.

3.2.1. Reagent Addition

A reagent addition step is described as the addition of a reagent (or mixture of reagents) in a constant volume to all wells on the plate. The control parameter is volume of the addition. In many cases, adequate mixing is achieved by the combination of the dispensing velocity and diffusion. In other case, agitation or mixing via up-and-down pipetting may be required. If reagent additions are performed by pipetting as opposed to noncontact dispensing, washing, or changing tips between plates may be required to avoid carryover.

3.2.2. Incubation

Incubation steps may be required for several purposes, including biochemical-reaction equilibrium, cell growth, scintillation proximity assay (SPA) bead settling. Control parameters are length of time and environmental conditions, commonly including temperature, humidity, and CO_2. From an automation perspective, there are many important details concerning incubation periods. What is the allowable range around the nominal incubation period? An assay with rapid-reaction kinetics might require tight control of the time period between starting the reaction and adding a stop reagent. Other reactions that go to completion may be primarily concerned with establishing a minimum incubation time. Whether or not plates can be stacked or lidded during incubation must be determined. In a fully automated system, a robotic incubator can be a complex and expensive part of the system. The interface between the incubator and the plate-handling robot is critical to ensure that the loading of one plate at a time, every few minutes, does not excessively perturb the environmental conditions that are being maintained. In contrast, with unit automation plates are loaded into the incubator in batches of a size appropriate for the particular assay. The principal concern in this case, is ensuring that if the incubator will be not just maintaining, but significantly changing the temperature of the plates, that the thermal mass of the plates loaded and the time to reach equilibrium is taken into account *(5)*.

3.2.3. Cell Plating

A specialized form of reagent dispensing, cell plating may require special provisions to avoid contamination, maintain uniform cell suspension and minimize temperature effects while out of the incubator. For example, developing a robust process for dispensing cells into 384-well microtiter plates was problematic. An 8-channel peristaltic-type dispenser had been commonly used for dispensing cell suspensions into 96-well plates. When the same equipment was used with 384-well plates, a small but unacceptable percentage of wells had trapped air bubbles at the bottom of the well. It was determined that if a

384-well pipettor was used to "pre-wet" the plates with media, the bubble problem was completely eliminated. As long as the bottom of the well was covered with media, the cell suspension would be drawn down to the bottom without trapping air.

This is a particularly good example of the power of decoupling steps using unit automation. Even though two steps (pre-wet and cell dispensing) were required, the overall operation was much more effective. One hundred 384-well plates could be loaded onto the 384-well pipetting workstation and the media pre-wetting operation could run unattended (in about 30 min) while the cells were being harvested. The cells could then be dispensed into the pre-wetted plates in another 30 min using a reagent dispenser.

3.2.4. Reaction Transfer

In some heterogeneous assay formats it is necessary to transfer the contents from a first plate to a different plate for further processing or detection. Enzyme-linked immunosorbent assay (ELISA), filter binding, and cell based assays that require removal of supernatant from the cell layer are just a few examples. The preferred methodology is to use a multichannel pipettor (96 or 384) to effect a simultaneous transfer from all wells of a plate. In addition, it is frequently important to minimize the time (or the variability of timing) across a given batch of plates.

3.2.5. Filtration

In HTS, filtration refers to a specialized unit operation used to separate bound and unbound assay components *(6)*. Filter plates and extraction equipment are available from numerous manufacturers (*see* Appendix A). Filter plates have a permeable membrane at the bottom of each well. When the plate is placed on a vacuum manifold, the well contents are pulled through the filter membrane and the permeate is separated from the filtrate. Generally, the permeate is waste and the filtrate is washed with buffer to remove remaining unbound material.

3.2.6. Plate Washing

Plate washing is required for many assay formats for a variety of reasons. Plate washing involves removing liquid from the wells and refilling with another liquid. All plate-washing operations are not alike. Some applications, such as coating plates with proteins, are simply concerned with effective removal of all excess residual coating. The addition and removal of the wash buffer can (and should be) quite vigorous, with relatively high flowrates to maximize throughput and leave as little residual liquid as possible.

In other cases, spent cell-culture media must be removed and replaced with fresh (or serum-containing media replaced with serum-free media). Some assay formats involve binding reactions where the unbound portion must be washed off. In other cases, cells may be loaded with dye *(7)*. At the end of the dye-loading period, the dye which has not been incorporated into the cells must be washed off. In any of these cell-washing applications, both the addition and aspiration must be carefully controlled to avoid damaging the cell layer. Liquid-flow rates, vacuum pressure, tip speed, tip height, and aspiration time are all variables that must be optimized for best results.

3.2.7. Plate Sealing

Frequently plates are sealed, either to provide containment of radiation or other potential hazards, or prevention of evaporation or contamination. Variables that determine the choice of seal stock include heat sealing vs adhesive seals, whether the plates will need to be unsealed, compatibility with solvents, suitability for low-temperature storage. There are also seals that can be pierced and resealed. Another important consideration is making sure that adhesive residue or loose seal edges will not cause problems for plate-handling equipment.

3.3. Signal Detection

The signal-detection unit operation is the key step where the biochemical activity is quantitatively measured. From an automation standpoint, whether the method employed is colorimetric absorbance, luminescence, SPA *(8)*, or any of the fluorescent formats is not as important as understanding the implications of throughput, cycle time, and signal stability. Reading a 384-well SPA plate on a 12 detector scintillation counter can take over 20 min per plate. But since this assay format is typically stable for 24–48 h, large batches of plates can be prepared and read on multiple counters over an extended period of time. Conversely, a cell-based chemiluminescent assay may need to be read within 30 min of lysing the cells *(9)*. In this case, it is necessary to restrict batch size to that which can be read within 30 min, or to utilize a reader with on-board reagent addition.

In the past, most detection systems have been based on Photo-Multiplier Tubes (PMTs). For those assay formats where signal collection time is significant (> 1–2 s) higher throughput is achieved by arranging multiple PMTs (up to 12) in parallel. The next advance involves switching from measuring individual wells to imaging the entire plate using a charge-coupled device (CCD) camera. This approach enables the reading of higher-density formats such as 1536-well plates, where reading one well at a time is not feasible.

The latest generation of CCD-based plate imaging systems have added to the advantage of unit automation. While these imagers are extremely sensitive and can have very high daily throughputs (100,000s of wells per day) they are also extremely expensive ($300k–500k). If one of these imagers is incorporated in a fully automated system, it cannot easily be shared by multiple assays that are in different phases of development, HTS, or follow-up. The workstation approach is much more amenable to shared utilization by a number of users.

4. Unit Automation in HTS

4.1. HTS is Different from Clinical Automation or SAR Support

One of the significant contrasts between the application of laboratory automation to HTS compared to clinical assays is the duration of the assay. In a clinical diagnostic laboratory, new test samples arrive on some periodic basis. The assay will be run perhaps for years, until a better assay replaces it. Similarly, screening in support of a medicinal chemistry Structure-Activity Relationship (SAR) effort deals with relatively few samples at a time, but may go on for months, even years in an iterative fashion.

In contrast, the objective of HTS is to screen hundreds of thousands of compounds for activity in an assay as quickly as possible, for only once the initial run is complete can the subsequent phases of confirmation and secondary assays take place. Because of this, a typical assay runs for only days, or at most weeks in an HTS lab. Consequently, there is a limited opportunity for assay level automation to "pay" for itself. In fact, if time is required to reconfigure, reprogram, and revalidate a fully automated system for each assay, considerable cost can be incurred. On the other hand, once the methodology for a unit operation is standardized and automated, it can be re-used over and over for a multitude of different assays.

5. Advantages of Unit Automation

5.1. Flexibility

As implied in the previous section, perhaps the greatest advantage of the unit-automation approach is flexibility. The building blocks that are the automated-unit operations can be combined in whatever order and quantity are required for a specific assay. **Figure 3** shows how assays can range from the simple, homogeneous, Add/Incubate/Read type to extremely complex, heterogeneous formats involving many steps, multiple incubations, and plate-to-plate transfers. A fully integrated system that has the capability to execute very complicated assay formats will require a great deal of space, sophisticated control algorithms, and equipment that can perform all the different unit operations.

Assay Complexity
From Simple......to Complex

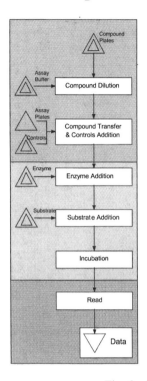

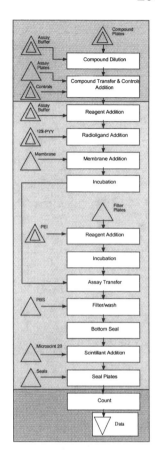

Fig. 3. Assays vary greatly in complexity.

5.2. System Reliability: Complex vs Simple and Serial vs Parallel

Robotic manipulators have become increasingly reliable and the software that controls them increasingly easy to use. However, the fact remains that in a fully automated assay system, the hardware and software that make up the robotic manipulator is, in many cases, the most complex portion of the entire system. Positional requirements involve moving plates several meters with an accuracy of tenths of millimeters, from hundreds of storage locations to dozens of instruments. On top of this is the complexity required of dynamic scheduling software to optimize utilization of both the robot and the instruments. Without a good dynamic scheduler, accrued lag time waiting on plates can add significant time to a method. The de facto result of this additional complexity is increased downtime, whether due to planned preventive maintenance or to unanticipated hardware or software failures.

Another approach uses many, simple, dedicated plate handlers to move plates from one instrument to the next. In this approach, each plate handler serves only one "source" and one "destination." While this greatly simplifies both the hardware and software demands, it also greatly increases the potential for downtime. It must be remembered that the reliability of a system is equal to the product of the reliability of individual components *(10,11)*. Thus, if there are 10 plate handlers in a system that each have an uptime of 99%, the expected uptime of the system is 0.99^{10} or only about 90%.

The unit automation approach avoids these additional opportunities for decreased reliability by omitting these elements entirely. Of course, this requires that people be available to move stacks of plates from one process step to the next, but especially with plates of increasing density (384, 1536, etc.) the number of operator actions required is minimized. In addition, when multiple workstations exist in a unit-automation environment, they can be used in parallel and provide redundancy in case of equipment failure.

5.3. Decoupling Facilitates Maximal Thruput

A significant advantage of unit automation is the ability to utilize available equipment to optimize thruput for a given assay *(12)*. For example, a colorimetric absorbance plate reader can read more than two hundred 96-well plates in 1 h. For a simple enzymatic assay with short incubation times, it might be desirable to team four 96 well pipettors (at a rate of 50 plates/h each) performing the compound transfer operation and be able to easily run 1200 96 well plates in an 8-h shift. Conversely, a cell-based ELISA might use the same plate reader, but be limited to 200 plates a day due to cell culture or plate washing capacity and thus only need one 96-well pipettor. In the fully automated approach, some fixed amount of capacity for each unit operation is dedicated to an assay system. This has the inevitable result of less than optimal thruput for straightforward assays or substantial underutilization of capacity at some steps for more complicated assays. The Gantt charts shown in **Tables 1–3** portray the flow of batches in a typical biochemical SPA. These charts illustrate not only the power of parallel processing, but also how miniaturization of assays into higher-density formats (96 to 384) dramatically reduces the number of operator interventions required.

In the assay illustrated in the Gantt charts, counting is performed in a single large batch. This is accomplished by a "workstation" (shown in **Fig. 4**) that is made up of other workstations. Three Wallac Microbeta Trilux scintillation

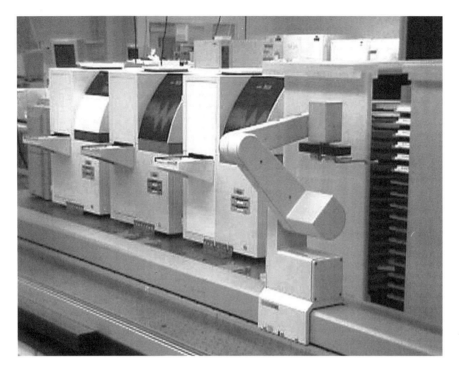

Fig. 4. Scintillation counting workstation.

counters are fed by an ORCA plate-handling robot from carousels that can hold up to 400 plates. This approach eliminates the need to load a batch of 16 plates every 2 h and maximally utilizes both the plate handling robot and the counters. By decoupling preparation of plates from counting, plates can be prepared in batch fashion in a very short period of time and counting can continue unattended through the night.

5.4. Independent Workstations Minimize Impact of New Instruments, Technologies

HTS is a rapidly evolving discipline *(13)*. Much of the equipment currently offered by leading instrument manufacturers was not even available three years ago *(see* Appendix B). New advances in miniaturized liquid handling, higher density plate formats, new detection technologies, proprietary reagent systems optimized for specialized detection platforms and other changes are continually emerging *(14)*.

Table 1
96-Well Plates, 400 Compound Plates/d

Step	Equipment	Batches	9:00	9:30	10:00	10:30	11:00	11:30	12:00	12:30	13:00	13:30	14:00	14:30	15:00	15:30	**Day 2** 8:00	8:30
Compound dilution	8-channel dispenser	16 × 25	1–4	5–8	9–12	13–16												
Compound transfer	96-well pipettor	8 × 50		1	3	5	7											
	96-well pipettor			2	4	6	8											
Substrate addition	8-channel dispenser	16 × 25			1–4	5–8	9–12	13–16										
Enzyme addition	8-channel dispenser	16 × 25				1–4	5–8	9–12	13–16									
Incubation	90 min																	
Stop/capture/bead addition	8-channel dispenser	16 × 25							1–4	5–8	9–12	13–16						
Plate sealing	Plate sealer	16 × 25								1–4	5–8	9–12	13–16					
Incubation	3–24 h																	
Count	Scintillation counters	1 × 400													1			1
Compounds tested	**32,000**																	
Stacker loads	**48**																	
Operator actions	**89**																	
Attended duration	**5 h**																	

384-Well Plates, 400 Compound Plates/d

Step	Equipment	Batches	9:00	9:30	10:00	10:30	11:00	11:30	12:00	12:30	13:00	13:30	14:00	14:30	15:00	15:30	Day 2 8:00	8:30	9:00
Compound dilution	8-channel dispenser	24 × 25	1–4	9–12	17–20														
	8-channel dispenser		5–8	13–16	21–24														
Compound transfer	96-well pipettor	15 × 40		1	5	9	13												
	96-well pipettor			2	6	10	14												
	96-well pipettor			3	7	11	15												
	96-well pipettor			4	8	12													
Substrate addition	8-channel dispenser	6 × 25			1 2 3	4 5 6													
Enzyme addition	8-channel dispenser	6 × 25				1 2 3	4 5 6												
Incubation	90 min																		
Stop/capture/bead addition	8-channel dispenser	6 × 25							1 2 3 4 5 6										
Plate sealing	Plate sealer	6 × 25								1 2 3 4 5 6									
Incubation	3–24 h																		
Read	Scintillation counters	1 × 150													1			1	

Compounds tested	48,000
Stacker loads	51
Operator actions	64
Attended duration	4.75 h

Table 3
384-Well Assay Plates, 150 384-Well Compound Plates/d

Step	Equipment	Batches	9:00	9:30	10:00	10:30	11:00	11:30	12:00	12:30	13:00	13:30	14:00	14:30	15:00	15:30	Day 2 8:00	8:30	9:00
Compound dilution	8-channel dispenser	6 × 25	1–3	4–6															
Compound transfer	384-well pipettor	6 × 25		1 2	3 4 5 6														
Substrate addition	8-channel dispenser	6 × 25			1 2 3	4 5 6													
Enzyme addition	8-channel dispenser	6 × 25				1 2 3	4 5 6												
Incubation	90 min																		
Stop/capture/bead addition	8-channel dispenser	6 × 25						1 2 3	4 5 6										
Plate sealing	Plate sealer	6 × 25							1 2 3	4 5 6									
Incubation	3–24 h																		
Read	Scintillation counters	1 × 150														1	1		
Compounds tested	**48,000**																		
Stacker loads	**12**																		
Operator actions	**37**																		
Attended duration	**4.25 h**																		

The impact of incorporating any of these advancements in a fully integrated automated screening system can be significant. Conversely, by its very nature, the unit automation approach confines the impact of changes to the specific unit operation involved. Proof-of-principle experiments, pilot runs or side-by-side comparisons vs existing methodologies can be readily performed with minimal impact to ongoing operations.

5.5. Incremental Capacity Additions Possible

Another significant advantage to the unit automation approach is the ability to add capacity in an incremental fashion. Capacity can be managed independently for each unit operation. Cycle time for a given unit operation can be measured. Cycle time multiplied by the number of workstations that can perform that operation, along with an estimate of utilization, results in the capacity (total throughput) for that unit operation. If a shortfall in capacity exists, it can be increased either by improvements that reduce cyle time, increasing utilization or, if neither of these are feasible, by adding another workstation. Conversely, in a fully integrated approach, adding capacity may very well require the addition of another complete system.

5.6. Access to Automation for Assay Development and Follow-Up

While the HTS timeline may only be days or weeks, both assay development and follow-up phases typically last for months *(15)*. The unit automation approach allows equal access to the same capabilities throughout all phases of a project. In the fully automated approach, unless a system is dedicated to a specific assay format, it will very likely be reconfigured after each HTS target.

6. Conclusions

Whether an HTS laboratory decides to utilizes workstation automation, fully integrated systems, or a combination of both approaches can be a matter of philosophy or culture, as much as technology or economics. In any case, the principals described in this chapter can be applied. The key points to remember are:

- Automate the process, not the assay. If an automated system is designed around the needs of a particular assay, the probability that it will have to be modified for subsequent assays is substantially increased. Instead, focus on the processes used in the operations to design systems that are assay independent.
- Identifying unit operations is key. The most important component of process-based automation design is breaking the process down into generic unit operations that can be utilized for a wide variety of assay formats. Once unit operations become the focus, improvements in methodologies, capacity, cycle time, and cost will benefit any assay that utilizes those particular unit operations.
- Standardize until it hurts...but be flexible. This seemingly contradictory statement is a powerful tool for prioritization. By standardizing wherever possible, on

equipment or methodologies, you can reserve flexibility for those occasions where it really matters. Standardization promotes incremental improvements, greater familiarity, fewer errors, and reduced learning curve.

- Look for the bottlenecks. The unit operation approach makes it easier to examine processes to determine where the true bottlenecks reside. Focusing resources on the bottleneck, whether to investigate improved methodologies or to add capacity, is the only way to improve the overall output of the system. Improvements in other areas will not result in benefit if a bottleneck in another area prevents their utilization.

- Remember the bottom line. We're not in the automation business; we're not even in the HTS business. We're in the business of drug discovery. A rapidly changing, continuously evolving enterprise, where tremendous sums are spent and failure and success cannot be evaluated until years down the road. Because of this, return on investment (ROI) or other financial payback calculations can't be utilized as easily as in other ventures where automation is frequently applied. This reality increases the importance of delivering the right automation solutions for the right problems.

References

1. Sills, M. A. (1997) Integrated robotics vs. task-oriented automation. *J. Biomol. Screening* **2,** 137–138.
2. Banks, M. (1997) High throughput screening using fully integrated robotic screening. *J. Biomol. Screening* **2,** 133–135.
3. Hopp, W. and Spearman, M. (1996) *Factory Physics*. Irwin, Chicago, IL.
4. Menke, K. (1999) Laboratory Automation: An Industrial Engineering Approach. International Symposium on Laboratory Automaion and Robotics 1999, Boston, MA.
5. Tanner, A. Helpful hints to manage edge effects of cultured cells for high throughput screening. Corning Cell Culture Application and Technical Notes. http://www.scienceproducts.corning.com/technical/an_hintsedgeeffecthts.pdf (18 Feb. 2001).
6. The Multiscreen Guide to Filtration Based Enzyme Assays MultiScreen Method. Millipore Lit. No. MM021.
7. Miller, T. R., et al. (1999) Antagonist affinity by FLIPR assay. *J. Biomol. Screening* **4,** 249–258.
8. Bosworth, N. and Towers, P. (1989) Scintillation proximity assay, *Nature* **341,** 167–168.
9. Luciferase Assay System (rev. 5/2000) Technical Bulletin No. 281, Promega Corporation, http://www.promega.com/tbs/TB281/tb281.pdf (19 Feb. 2001).
10. Lipson, C. and Sheth, N. (1973) Analysis of systems, in *Statistical Design and Analysis of Engineering Experiments*, McGraw-Hill, New York, NY, pp. 345–355.
11. Brandt, D. (1998) Core system model: understanding the impact of reliability on high-throughput screening systems. *Drug Discovery Today* **3(2),** 61–68.

12. Oldenburg, K. (1999) Automation basics: robotics vs. workstations. *J. Biomol. Screening* **4,** 53–56.
13. Divers, M. (1999) What is the future of high throughput screening? *J. Biomol. Screening* **4,** 177–178.
14. Fox, S., et al. (1999) High throughput screening for drug discovery: continually transitioning into new technology. *J. Biomol. Screening* **4,** 183–186.
15. Valler, M. and Green, D. (2000) Diversity screeening versus focussed screening in drug discovery. *Drug Discovery Today* **5(7),** 286–293.

Appendix A
Manufacturers of Filter Plates Used in High Throughput Screening

Manufacturer/Product	Website
Corning/Filter Plates	http://www.scienceproducts.corning.com/
Millipore/Multiscreen™	http://www.millipore.com/
Packard Biosciences/OmniFilter™	http://www.packardbioscience.com
PerkinElmer Wallac/Acro Well, Harvest Plate	http://www.wallac.com/
Whatman Polyfiltronics®/UniFilters™	http://www.whatman.com/

Appendix B
HTS Workstations Introduced Since 1998

Manufacturer	Model	Type	Date
Tecan	Polarion	Fluorescence	1998
Labsystems™	Fluoroskan Ascent FL™	Multilabel	1998
Packard	MultiPROBE® II	Pipettor	1998
Packard	PlateTrak®	Pipettor	1998
Tomtec	Quadra96/384®	Pipettor	1998
Hudson Control Group	PlateCrane™	Plate Handler	1998
Hudson Control Group	PlateSilo™	Plate Handler	1998
Packard	PlateStak	Plate Handler	1998
Amersham Pharmacia	LEADseeker Generation 1	Plate Imager	1998
Labsystems™	Nepheloskan™ Ascent™	Turbidity	1998
Titertek	MAP Series	Washer	1998
Tri Continent	Encore 2000™	Washer	1998
Labsystems™	Multiskan™ Ascent™	Absorbance	1999
Titertek®	Multidrop 384™ with S60 Stacker	Dispenser	1999
Molecular Dynamics®	Typhoon 8600	Gel Scanner	1999
Tecan	Ultra	Multilabel	1999
Wallac™	1420 VICTOR ^{2}™	Multilabel	1999
Cartesian Technologies	PegaSys™ 320	Pipettor	1999
Cartesian Technologies	PixSys™ 3200	Pipettor	1999
Cartesian Technologies	PixSys™ 5500	Pipettor	1999
Tecan	GenMate	Pipettor	1999
Amersham Pharmacia	LEADseeker Generation 2	Plate Imager	1999
Tecan	PowerWash 384	Washer	1999
Tri Continent	Multiwash II™	Washer	1999

Tri Continent	Multiwash Advantage	Washer	1999
Packard	Alphaquest®	Fluorescence	2000
Wallac™	Flite	Fluorescence	2000
Packard	Fusion®	Multilabel	2000
Tecan	Genios	Multilabel	2000
Tecan	Safire	Multilabel	2000
Wallac™	1420 VICTOR V™	Multilabel	2000
Beckman Coulter	Biomek® FX	Pipettor	2000
Labsystems™	Wellpro 384	Pipettor	2000
Packard	MultiPROBE® HTS	Pipettor	2000
Tecan	TeMo-96	Pipettor	2000
Tecan	Genesis NPS	Pipettor	2000
Tomtec	Quadra3	Pipettor	2000
Tomtec	QuadraPlus®	Pipettor	2000
Amersham Pharmacia	LEADseeker Generation 3	Plate Imager	2000
Applied Biosystems	Northstar™	Plate Imager	2000
Wallac™	ViewLux™	Plate Imager	2000
Labsystems™	Wellwash 384	Washer	2000
Tomtec	Quadra-Wash® 96/384	Washer	2000

12

Fully Automated Screening Systems

Seth Cohen and Robert F. Trinka

1. Selecting the Hardware
1.1. Introduction

As a scientist or manager involved with high throughput screening (HTS), you have a wide range of options when selecting the degree of automation to support your discovery efforts. You will want to think about your anticipated needs 2–4 yr (or more) into the future and whether those projected needs will require a fully automated system.

Initially, many organizations use individual workstations for pipetting, incubating, mixing, washing, dispensing, plate reading, etc., with lab technicians moving the plates from station to station. This is simpler and requires less capital expense than a fully automated robotic system. The disadvantage with the workstation-based laboratory is that the processing of the assay and the overall plate throughput is very dependent on the lab technicians themselves. The results of the assay can vary significantly according to the attention to detail given by the laboratory technicians, and overall throughput also can vary significantly according to the staffing levels and the technicians' interest in processing the microplates as accurately, quickly, and efficiently as possible.

As throughput requirements and laboratory budgets increase, the disadvantages of manual workstations compel users to consider fully automated robotic systems. Fortunately, some types of fully automated robotic system are very flexible, can use many of the manual workstation instruments that you are already using in your laboratory, and allow the individual workstations in the fully automated system to be upgraded in the future as these devices are improved.

The degree to which you automate your laboratory will depend on many factors, including your throughput requirements and how this will grow in the

From: *Methods in Molecular Biology, vol. 190: High Throughput Screening: Methods and Protocols*
Edited by: W. P. Janzen © Humana Press Inc., Totowa, NJ

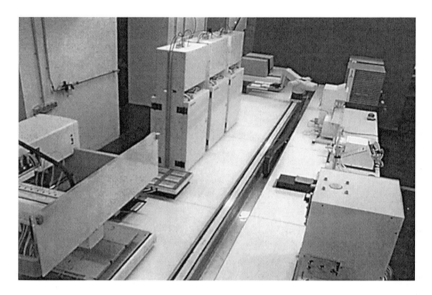

Fig. 1. Example of a fully automated high throughput screening system.

future and the amount of money that can be allocated to automation. A picture of a fully automated robotic system is shown in **Fig. 1**.

Some of the advantages of fully automated robotic systems or HTS include:

1. Assay steps performed consistently from run to run, independent of the operator.
2. Data and compound identification can be automatically tracked through the primary screen, confirmatory assays, and secondary screens with no errors.
3. Some types of fully automated robotic systems will run unattended continuously 24 h per day, 7 d/wk to provide maximum plate throughput.
4. Flexible robotic systems can run many different types of assays with no change-over time or learning curve.

The mantra of virtually every HTS laboratory is flexibility, reliability, and reproducibility. When considering various types of equipment, be sure to fully investigate the equipment and the vendor to make sure that they offer the best of these requirements. Reliability can be determined by checking with other users and investigating the equipment yourself. Reproducibility can be measured by performing standard evaluation tests, either within your department, by the vendor, or by a third party such as another user of the instrument.

1.2. Your Future Needs and HTS Trends: Divining The Future

Certainly it is very difficult to predict your future needs, as well as future trends in the industry, but you want your fully automated HTS system to be as compatible as possible with the methods and protocols that you'll likely use in the future. Some trends can be identified and are listed below. The key word for any system, however, is "flexibility". In order to protect your investment as well as ensure the continued throughput in your department, you need equipment that is flexible so it can be adapted to your future needs.

Some of the continuing trends in high throughput screening are:

1. Increased density of microplates;
2. Newer detection technologies including various imaging devices for fluorescence and luminescence assays; and
3. Movement away from assays which require separation steps such as washing and filtering, and away from radioactive assays.

By definition, flexible, fully automated robotic systems are reprogrammable and can easily adapt to new assays and new or upgraded instruments required for the assays. Some of the things that you'll want to do to improve the implementation of the fully automated system are:

1. Involve the users in your laboratory to define the system requirements and select the vendor.
2. Gather information from other users and vendor references regarding the desired features of various systems, things that they would do differently, and other recommendations. Experienced users usually have suggestions that are gained through trial and error, and you want to minimize your trials and errors.
3. It will be helpful to have frequent meetings possibly weekly, as the members of the task force report on various assignments to collect your internal needs and report on the investigation of various possible vendors.
4. Remember that the time spent reviewing the system and vendor-selection criteria BEFORE placing an order will be well spent and give you a more optimum robotic system to meet your needs.

1.3. What to Do Before Placing the Order

1.3.1. Defining Your Needs

The process of defining your needs and selecting the appropriate equipment and vendors can be a time-consuming, tedious process, and the temptation is to treat this as an interruption to your other job responsibilities. If you will take the time to define your needs and specify that the equipment must first be tested to meet those requirements before shipment to your laboratory, you will save yourself considerable headache and heartache after the equipment arrives at your laboratory.

1.3.2. Check the Details and Fine Print

Define the system acceptance criteria and get the vendor's policy on who pays for the transportation, site installation, and training. Most robotic systems are sold FOB the factory, although the vendor will usually prepay and bill the freight. Many vendors have an additional charge for the time and expenses for the installation engineers to install the robotic system in your laboratory. It is usually difficult for either organization to estimate this cost, and most users don't like the open-ended nature of this type of billing.

Some vendors include the cost of installation in the overall price of the robotic system and this is better for you. First, you are not subject to additional invoices over which you have no control and which can be difficult to justify to your management, particularly if you didn't have enough money in the budget to cover these expenses. And secondly, vendors that include it in the overall price are confident that the system will be installed and accepted by the user well within the budgeted time. This tells you that the supplier is more confident of the successful operation of the robotic system as soon as it is installed.

Note that it is quite common for the vendor's delivery to slip. This is obviously can be a serious problem, particularly if you are on a tight time schedule to begin actual screens. You can reduce the chance of this happening by thoroughly investigating the vendor's references, verifying that your fully automated system is very similar to previous systems that have been delivered on time, and possibly writing into the purchase contract a penalty for late delivery.

1.3.3. Training is Very Important

You will also want to have as many people as possible trained on the robotic system. With personnel turnover and transfers, you want a pool of people who are trained and can operate the robotic system. The first people to be trained should be those who: 1) have operated a robotic system before, or 2) will be operating the system, or 3) have a good mechanical aptitude. There are many details and nuances in the operation of fully automated systems, and you will find your organization relying heavily on the supplier's manuals and training program. Many fully automated robotic systems will use third-party peripherals for dispensing, detecting, or other specialized functions, and those devices may have their own manuals and training programs.

Because there are many details to learn in order to operate and use the fully automated system, you will find a 'catch 22' with the factory training. Of course, people must have some training before they can operate the robotic system, but they will learn the most after they have had some experience with the system. This is because after a few months of operation, they will have developed an appreciation for why some information is of value and they will also ask questions specific questions that might have been omitted by the trainer. You will find that the best solution is to have training when the robotic system is installed (or before), but also have a follow-up training session 3–12 mo after installation. This will be invaluable as a refresher course and you will find that your team will make a quantum leap in their understanding of the automation system after the second training course.

1.3.4. Include an Unattended Run in the Acceptance Criteria

As part of your purchase order, you should include an acceptance criteria that includes at least one 12 h (or longer) unattended run in your laboratory using all peripherals. Although you should also insist on an acceptance test at the vendor's factory before shipping, you should still insist on an acceptance test in your laboratory to make sure that any damage that might have occurred during shipping is found and that the fully automated system is properly installed in your laboratory.

1.4. What to Do Before Your Robotic System Arrives

After you have selected the vendor and placed the order, there are still many things that you can and should be doing before the system arrives. The temptation is to get back to your work, whether on the bench or in the office, and let the vendor 'do their thing.' In reality, you have considerable work to perform to get ready for the equipment installation.

Users who are part of a large site will usually have their site engineering departments assist in coordinating the various installation steps with the vendor. This will include having the appropriate utilities brought to the proper place in the lab so they will connect to those on the automated system. Experienced vendors will have specifications that you can actually review before placing the order so you can evaluate the site-installation costs and put the appropriate amount into your budget.

The utilities can include electricity, computer connections, compressed air and vacuum, liquid drains, vapor recovery, etc. The vendor will be able to give you a drawing of the robotic system and the specific ratings (electrical amperage and voltage, for example) that the system will require.

You should begin writing your Standard Operating Procedures (SOPs) for the operation, calibration, and validation of the major third-party peripherals and the fully automated system as a whole. Unfortunately users commonly delay these details until after the robotic system arrives, but, at that point, you'll be busy trying to run your assays on the system, so the ideal time to begin researching and writing these documents is before the system is installed.

2. Assay Development for Fully Automated High Throughput Screens
2.1. Introduction

Development of assays which will be implemented on HTS systems in fully automated mode requires one to address the same issues as the development of the assay to be run in workstation or partially automated mode. Among these considerations are detection format, signal/noise window, assay chemistry, reproducibility, signal and reagent stability, compound concentration /presentation, assay artifacts, and overall assay quality (as quantified by such metrics as % CV or Z' factor *[1]*). Although these considerations are common to both fully automated and workstation approaches, often additional attention to several of them is required to implement the HTS on a fully automated system.

Fully automated systems may run the HTS for extended periods of time, some even completing the full screening library in a single run extending for more than a week. The stability of the reaction components (cells, enzymes, substrates, compounds) and the resulting signal often becomes a major focus of the assay-development effort. Bulk reagent preparation and storage conditions, as well as the storage capacity for assay consumables on the system, are also related issues. The stability of the complete assay is dependent on the combined stability of all components, therefore an understanding of the stability of all parts of the assay is required.

Specific examples of the development of fully automated HTS for cell-based and in vitro assays are described below. Issues that were critical to successful implementation of these assays as fully automated screens are discussed.

2.2. Cell-Based Assay

2.2.1. Introduction

The first example is a 384-well growth inhibition assay using a hypersensitive strain of the yeast *Candida albicans*. The goal of the HTS was to identify growth inhibitory antifungal agents. This microbial growth assay was originally developed for a workstation assay and later reconfigured to run on an automated system in fully automated mode. The assay involves a 20 µL dispense of a dilute (50 mOD_{600}) *C. albicans* culture in liquid growth media into a clear 384-well plate containing 5 µL of dilute screening compound dispensed previously by the compound dispensary and stored at –20°C in vacuum bags prior to the HTS. Control compounds are added and the plates are incubated with lids at 30°C. Final assay conditions are 25 µL/well, 5 µM test compounds, <1% dimethyl sulfoxide (DMSO). In the workstation version of the HTS, the cells were diluted from an overnight culture, grown out for 2 h with shaking, rediluted to 50 mOD_{600} and immediately dispensed into up to 80 microtiter plates using a Labsystems Multidrop 8-channel peristaltic dispenser with a sterilized dispensing cassette. Control compounds were added manually with an 8-channel pipettor prior to the cell addition. Following cell addition a zero time read at OD_{600} was acquired with a microplate reader with plate stacker.

The plates were then lidded and incubated at 30°C for 18–20 h prior to the final OD_{600} read.

2.2.2. Procedure

The goal was to convert the assay to run on the automated system. The assay plates would still be loaded onto the system already containing the test compounds, however now the control and cell additions, the incubations and the reads would all be processed on the system. The robotic system that we used has a capacity for 216 plates in its 4 incubators, so we targeted 216 plates (75,000 tests) as our desired capacity for each HTS run. Approximately 4 L of cells would be required to source the 216 plates. One major change in the method necessitated by the switch to full automation was the requirement for the cells to be dispensed over a long period of time. In the workstation version, 80 plates could be dispensed in as little as 30 min (less than half of 1 doubling time for this culture at room temperature.) In a 216 plate full automation run, the time to dispense the cells would take almost 18 h. Using the original workstation SOP, the cells would continue to grow following dilution into the room temperature media. Therefore at the time of the dispense into the assay plates, there would be increasing cells, leading to an inconsistent and insensitive assay. Continuously providing dilute cells to the system (for example, every hour) would be impractical over the 18 h necessary to process all 216 plates and increase the risk of contamination.

Since online refrigeration was available on the system, we attempted to determine the stability and sensitivity of the strain held at 4–6°C for extended periods prior to dispense into the assay plate. We addressed a number of growth-related issues including the growth rate (if any) of cells held in the refrigerated reservoir and the incubation time necessary for the cells grown out from this storage condition. We also determined the viable cell number as a function of time held in the refrigerated reservoir. If the cold storage altered the sensitivity of the strain to inhibitory compounds, it might invalidate this approach to the assay.

To prepare the cells, the workstation protocol was followed from the overnight cell growth until the final dilution of the cells into the room temperature media. The dilute cell suspension was then placed in the refrigerator for 2 h prior to the initiation of the dispense to the assay plates. Viable cell counts were determined by plating out dilutions of the cell suspension at various times included just after the final dilution into the room temperature media (Time 0) and at numerous subsequent time points out to 40 h at 4–6°C. To our surprise, the cell number and viability remained constant during the full 40 h of the

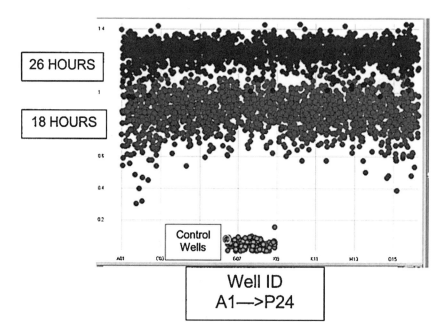

Fig. 2. Growth of cells in a 384-well microplate over 18 and 26 h.

experiment, suggesting that this method could be used to maintain a consistent cell number for dispensing throughout the course of the automated HTS.

2.2.3. Results

Although the viable cell counts remained constant, because of previous experiences, we suspected that the refrigerated cells may experience a greater lag in growth by the automation method compared with the workstation version in which the cells were immediately dispensed from the room temperature media. In the workstation method, the cells reached their maximum growth in the wells following 18–20 hours at 30°C. We set up a series of experiments on the automated system which varied the incubation time of the cells from 18–40 h. **Figure 2** shows these results.

Compared with the previously developed workstation HTS (manual), the time required for completion of cell growth in the wells was extended by approx 8 h, requiring an extension of the incubation time from 18 h to 26 h. This finding suggested that the cells experience a prolonged lag phase before initiation of growth and division when held at the lower temperature.

One key validation issue was the sensitivity of the strain following prolonged storage at the refrigerated temperature and comparison of these results with the Minimal Inhibitory Concentrations (MIC) determined by the workstation

Table 1
Comparison Between Manual (Workstation) and Full Automation Minimum Inhibitory Concentrations (MICs) for a Range of Antifungal Compounds

Test compounds	Manual MICs µg/mL	Automation MICs µg/mL
Tunicamycin	0.81	1.79
4-nitroquinilone	0.02	0.05
Cerulenin	0.20	0.20
Amphotericin B	0.20	0.28
Fluconazole	0.10	0.10
Ketaconazole	0.03	0.07
Nystatin	20.80	12.48

method. A panel of known antifungal agents with different modes of action were prepared by serial dilution and included with the uniformity plates during the robotic validation runs. MIC determinations (**Table 1**) determined that no significant change was observed for any of the compounds tested by the changes made in the SOP to accommodate the automated version of the assay.

2.2.4. Sterility

Sterility is an additional area of concern in the development of an automated version of an assay. Contamination of the cell reservoir or the assay plates could lead to false negative results. All possible sources of contamination including incubators, reagent-dispensing lines, pipeting canulas, and exposed surfaces were cleaned with 70% ethanol prior to and after each run. Special attention was paid to the handling of the compound plates. The room containing the system was monitored regularly using settling plates. The completed assay plates were disposed of promptly into the appropriate bio-waste bins and removed from the premises immediately.

2.3. Noncell-Based Assay

2.3.1. Introduction

Scintillation proximity assays (SPA) are a popular format for prosecuting kinase screens. In the following example, the goal was to develop a 384-well SPA assay for a purified kinase enzyme. The enzyme phosphorylated a small peptide substrate, which was biotinylated to allow for capture to Streptavidin-coated SPA beads. The benchtop assay was optimized for the Km's for the two substrates, ATP and the peptide. The amount of Streptavidin beads and ^{33}P-ATP were also optimized to provide the best signal/background window. The reaction time-course studies suggested that the reaction was linear for at least 6 h *(2)*.

2.3.2. Procedure

The automated system that was used for this HTS was designed specifically for SPA assays, but isotopic assays are widely performed on fully automated systems that also run nonisotopic assays. The only additional equipment that is required accommodates the 'hot' or radioactive compounds and detects the assay results. This particular fully automated robotic system consists of a central robot on a 3-foot track; two high-capacity temperature controlled incubators; a 96–384 channel pippetor; three Multidrop® 384 dispensers and two Wallac® 12-detector Microbeta Trilux® readers for detection of the SPA signal. The plates and datafiles are tracked using a bar-code reader on the system. Due to the relatively long time required to read the SPA signal (15–>30 min/plate) the system throughput is typically limited by the number of readers.

Because of the long plate-reading time, in order to achieve the maximum throughput (plates/d), the system should operate as close to 24 h/d as possible. The initial automation attempt used preformatted 384-well DMSO compound plates already containing controls in the appropriate wells. To these plates, 15 µL of substrate buffer and 10 µL of enzyme were added to the compound plate using two of the Multidrops. Following incubation of 90 min at room temperature, a stirred stop solution containing Strepavidin beads was dispensed into the plates using a third Multidrop.

The beads were allowed to settle for 8 h prior to the read. The read for the first plate through the system was nearly 10 h after the start of the screen. The read time of 60 s/well limited us to about 4 plates/h using both detectors. To validate the automation, a uniformity run on the system was performed. The method used would process one plate per hour for 24 h. Enzyme and substrate solutions were dispensed from a refrigerated cabinet and the solutions in the Multidrop tubing were automatically withdrawn back into the chilled reservoir after each dispense. This kept the reagents in a chilled environment as long as possible. Modern peristaltic dispensers have commands to empty the lines and reprime after each dispense.

2.3.3. Results

Figure 3 shows the results of this first 24-plate uniformity run. The kinase activity appears to be reduced as a function of time, giving consistent (and expected) signal for the first 3–4 h but dropping off steadily. By the 16th plate, the activity is barely detectable above the background. This result suggested that one or more of the assay components was not stable during the assay. The

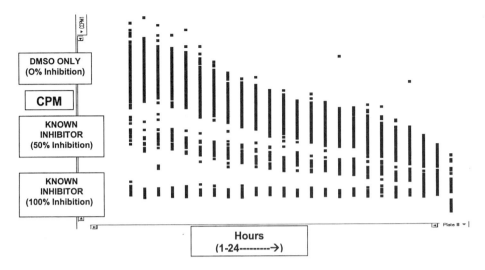

Fig. 3. Results of a 24 microplate uniformity run.

likely suspect was the enzyme. All previous stability studies had been done with the enzyme stored on ice.

On the system, a small refrigeration unit is used to hold and chill the enzyme to maintain its stability. Using temperature monitors, it was determined that the refrigerator was not holding temperature to specifications (2–6°C) but was in fact fluctuating up to 12°C. The uniformity plates were run again. This time the enzyme and substrate reservoirs were placed directly in an ice bucket next to the Multidrop dispenser. The bucket was covered to reduce the rate of the ice melting. This time the assay gave high and consistent signal for the full run of 24 h continuously. (**Fig. 4**).

The refrigeration system was adjusted and the HTS was run again, paying close attention to the monitoring of the refrigerator temperature. This illustrates the importance of performing a validation run before running the actual screen and potentially wasting valuable compounds and reagents.

3. Other Topics

3.1. Validation

3.1.1. Introduction

A key step in the commissioning of a fully automated HTS is the validation of the system. Obviously if the automation system hasn't been validated, then you can't rely on the data generated. So validation becomes first and foremost the most important task after system installation and acceptance from the ven-

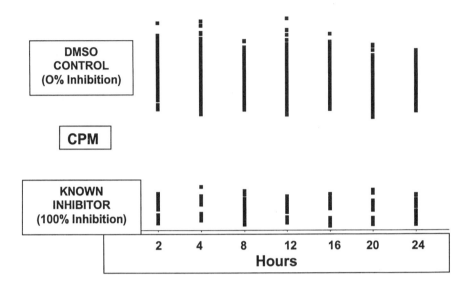

Fig. 4. Results of the assay using properly chilled enzyme.

dor. Some people may be tempted to take shortcuts, but the most methodical, although sometimes not the fastest method, is to first validate each instrument by itself, then validate the system as a whole.

3.1.2 What You Can Do Before the Fully Automated System Arrives

While you are waiting for your fully automated system to arrive, you can begin preparing for the system validation. Now is a good time to contact each of the suppliers for any of the instruments that will be part of the automation system. Ask for the recommended maintenance, calibration, and validation procedures for each of the devices that will be part of your fully automated system. In addition, find out what training is offered and recommended. You can decide whether to take the training before the system is installed or afterwards, but remember that it virtually always takes longer than anticipated to start running assays, so it's better to do things before installation than afterwards if you want to stay as close to schedule as possible.

3.1.3. System Validation

The steps of validation include first verifying that both the hardware and software were installed properly to become a qualified system *(3)*. Then a method is performed and validated. Finally, complete validation is achieved when the suitability of the system is assessed for your specific purposes. All of these steps must be documented and on file at the automation system for fast future reference in case there is a quality audit or if there is any question about the validation procedure *(4)*.

Thus, in order to validate the automation system, you will first request and receive any information from all of the suppliers of any third-party instruments or devices for any validation information and procedures for their instruments. You must run these tests to verify that the instrument is performing within allowable tolerances. Keep the test procedures and results of these tests in your files. (Remember that you'll want to periodically verify that the instrument is operating within allowable ranges, so you'll need to periodically run the required procedures. Each instrument vendor should recommend how frequently their device should be verified to be operating properly.)

After validating the operation of each device, you are prepared to select a method and run it on the automation system. You must compare the results with those performed by a previously validated method and verify that the results are within allowable tolerances. When the results are comparable, you have now validated a method on the automated system. Document the method and results and file it with the previous validation results.

The final step is to list the types of assays that can be properly performed on the automated system. When all of these steps have been completed, you have validated your automation system.

Although the validation steps can be time-consuming *(5)*, it is absolutely critical that they be performed precisely and correctly. You cannot begin to have confidence in the data generated by the automated system if you have not verified that the automation system is capable of producing accurate data. As scientists and technologists, we all recognize the importance of these basic steps before running actual assays. The investment in reagents, compounds and time is too great to risk it on running the assay on a nonvalidated automated system.

When testing liquid dispensing or pipetting accuracy, fluorescein or tartrazine are commonly used because the strength of the fluorescence reading is directly proportional to the amount in the plate well *(6,7)*. Your instrument vendors will be able to recommend other materials and procedures for validating the operation of their products.

3.2. System Troubleshooting

3.2.1. Introduction

Troubleshooting an HTS robotic system requires a systematic analysis of the observed deviation and a careful consideration of the possible causes. It is a two-step process: first establish where the problem is, then determine how to correct it. When analyzing a problem on the automated system, you must first determine if the problem is with the chemistry of the assay itself, or if the cause is with the automated system. Regardless of the cause, you must work to isolate it and then develop a solution. You will find that you must examine every step, including rechecking reagents and plasticware, verifying that instruments are still within calibration, etc.

3.2.2. Random and Systematic Errors

Sources of error might be systematic or random. Systematic error causes a general shift of the data, which is easier to observe than random errors, which can affect one or a few data points, but then disappear as quickly as it appeared. Systematic errors might have either mechanical or biological/chemical causes, but by isolating and testing each individual possible cause, the source of the problem can eventually be found.

Random errors are much more difficult to find, but the troubleshooter can take heart that most random errors have a mechanical cause that hasn't progressed enough to be consistent enough to become a systematic problem.

For example, incorrect readings that seem to be in one part of a micro plate more often than others might be due to occasional large variances in reagent dispensing, uneven heating during incubation, inaccurate plate reading, etc., all which would point to a mechanical component that is beginning to fail. In order to find the cause of the deviation, you will be required to carefully observe the movement of the various mechanical devices in the robotic system as well as devise experiments to test the various subcomponents.

Experienced users of automated systems keep a log at the system of everything unusual that is observed during any run. The log is just a simple listing of the following: Date, Time, What Was Observed, Any Action Taken, Who Reported It, etc. Forms should be pre-printed with these headings (make any changes to this suggestion) and hole punched so they can be kept in a three-ring notebook binder with the other manuals at the robotic system. Make sure that any unusual observations are written down. This error log history will be invaluable in trying to identify potential causes of problems.

3.2.3. Possible Problems That Might Occur

1. Dispensing of reagents.
   a. Temperature-sensitive reagents warm up waiting to be dispensed into the plate.
   b. Reagents that are suspensions (cells, beads, etc.) settle while waiting to be dispensed.

    c. The dispensing device doesn't dispense the same volume to each of the wells.

    d. The reagent coats or reacts with the inside surface of the fluid path, possibly losing some of its chemical properties or gaining unwanted properties.

    e. Uneven dispensing can be caused by restricted flow in the fluid path, nonuniform pumping action, incomplete valve actuation, etc.

2. Heating/incubation.

    a. Edge effects: some wells receive more (or less) heat, CO_2, or humidity than other wells.

    b. Temperature, CO_2, or humidity control isn't precise enough, causing too much variation between plates.

3. Plate washing: Not consistent or inaccurate, either from well to well within a plate, or from plate to plate.

4. Reader calibration: The reader may have the wrong or incorrectly calibrated plate definition.

4. Summary

A fully automated system is one of the most valuable tools available for HTS. However, proper sourcing, installation and operation of an automated system requires a thorough inventory of your needs and a strong attention to detail in the implementation and operation.

As you could see from the examples, assays can usually be transferred to an automated robotic system with minimum changes. However details must be reviewed to assure that the results will be consistent within a run and as compared to the same assay performed manually on the bench or on workstations.

Validation is a crucial element to assure that the integrated system and the individual components are operating within their designated tolerances.

References

1. Zhang, J., Chung, T. D. Y., and Oldenburg, K. R. (1999) A simple statistical parameter for use in evaluation and validation of high throughput screening assays. *J. Biomol. Screening* **4,** 67–73.

2. Cook, N. D. (1996) Scintillation proximity assay: a versatile high throughput screening technology. *Drug Discovery Today* **1,** 287.

3. Swartz, M. and Krull, I. (1997) *Analytical Method Development and Validation.* Marcel Dekker, Inc., New York, NY, p. 20.

4. Stanley, J. (1999) Development and Validation Guidelines for Automated Methods Proceedings of International Symposium of Laboratory Automation and Robotics, ISLAR, Hopkinton, MA.

5. Zick, F. and Fischer, M. J. (2000) Robotic and automated systems, in *The Pharmaceutical QC*, Proceedings of International Symposium of Laboratory Automation and Robotics, ISLAR, Hopkinton, MA.

6. Seybold, G., Gouterman, M., and Callis, J. (1969) Calorimetric, photometric and lifetime determinations of fluorescence yields of fluorescein dyes. *Photochem. Photobiol.* **9,** 229–242.
7. Haugland, R. (1996), *The Handbook of Fluorescent Probes and Research Chemicals, Sixth Edition.* Molecular Probes, Eugene, OR.

Other Suggested Resources

Although not specially referred to in this text, there are a number of publications that frequently print articles on fully automated systems for high throughput screening.

Journal of Biomolecular Screening, Society of Biomolecular Screening, Danbury CT. Publisher: Mary Ann Liebert, Inc., Larchmont, NY.

Proceedings: International Symposium of Laboratory Automation and Robotics, Zymark Corp., Hopkinton, MA (published yearly).

Journal of the Association of Laboratory Automation (JALA), Association for Laboratory Automation, Charlottesville, VA.

Associations

Association for Laboratory Automation, PO Box 800572, Charlottesville, VA 22908, www.labautomation.org

The Laboratory Robotics Interest Group (LRIG), 1730 West Circle Drive Martinsville, NJ 08836-2147, www.lab-robotics.org

Society for Biomolecular Screening, 36 Tamarack Avenue, #348, Danbury, CT 06811, www.SBSonline.org

13

Management and Maintenance of High Throughput Screening Systems

Barbara Hynd

1. Introduction

The object of all high throughput screening (HTS) laboratories is to provide the pharmaceutical research community with potentially active compounds rapidly and in the most cost effective manner possible. The most reliable way this can be achieved is by rigorous attention to the quality of the assays themselves, the quality of the compounds used, as well as the quality and condition of the equipment used. To effectively reach this goal all of the systems needed within the screening environment must function in a smooth, efficient manner. Since the complexity of the equipment used in screening labs is constantly increasing, the requirements for its continued maintenance are problems faced in all laboratories. An additional process that requires constant maintenance, but that is often forgotten, is management of personnel within the screening environment. This is, however, also an integral part of the efficient screening process.

In most companies HTS has evolved out of the research area and these groups have had to learn to adapt manufacturing principles for use in a research environment in order to become efficient. Since research laboratories do not have to conform to Food and Drug Administration (FDA) requirements as do the development and production laboratories, the concept of routine quality control has been alien to many that move into screening laboratories. Reliability has always been expected of laboratory equipment, but in research laboratories there was usually little impact if equipment was unavailable for a day or so. This situation is not acceptable in HTS since the whole premise is that nothing should stand in the way of the screens being run. Project timelines, which are set with the expectation that HTS is a fast process, can be adversely

From: *Methods in Molecular Biology, vol. 190: High Throughput Screening: Methods and Protocols*
Edited by: W. P. Janzen © Humana Press Inc., Totowa, NJ

affected if the equipment is unreliable or the screening assays are not robust and reproducible. Thus accuracy of equipment performance is a vital part of maintaining an efficient screening facility.

2. Equipment Requirements

The equipment found in HTS facilities varies from workstation like instrumentation to large multitasking robotic installations. All of these systems have evolved according to the requirements of the individual companies and their methods of working. Some laboratories only take a limited number of assay types as HTS and thus require a limited variety of instrumentation. Larger facilities may have the luxury of sufficient numbers of fully automated robotic platforms, which can be dedicated to individual assay types. There are also other groups intermediate to these two extremes who require as much flexibility in their screening repertoire as possible. All of these groups have the same core requirements: accuracy, precision robustness, and reproducibility, both for the equipment and the assays themselves. The equipment and support systems, discussed in this chapter, will be a representation of those commonly found in the chemical repository and assay throughput areas of an average HTS facility.

2.1. Chemical Repository

There is no current universally preferred format for a chemical repository and the maintenance methods depend on the equipment and format of the repository itself. The current storage methods depend on the library format and can range from storage as dry films in an inert atmosphere at $-80°C$ to storage at room temperature in dimethyl sulfoxide (DMSO). Universal acceptance of one set of conditions for compound storage has not yet occurred for a number of reasons. The main one is lack of adequate data as to which conditions are really optimal since degradation studies performed by individual companies have not been published. The cost of replacing existing storage facilities is also a major concern to company management and has to be balanced against the value of the existing library. The result of this is that each company has developed a compound handling system that is peculiar to their situation.

Irrespective of the system used, control of the environmental factors must be recorded either by manual logging of temperature, humidity, and oxygen levels or by continuous electronic monitoring. The latter method is the one of choice since it is less prone to error and can give accurate timing of adverse events. Most older, manual or semi-manual storage instrumentation can be retrofitted with fully automated recording and alarm devices at a nominal cost. Continuous charting of the collected data will give indications of some potential problems but should not preclude regular visual examinations of known problem areas such as seals and vents. In addition any robotic or mechanical component of the system must have a regular maintenance schedule set up and strictly adhered to (*see* equipment maintenance, **Subheading 4.**).

The quality control of any library, whatever the format, is very important and it is particularly advisable to have analytical checks done at regular intervals for any library that is held in a liquid format. The chemical composition of the compounds should be confirmed prior to addition to the library and the method used should be routine for the analytical services used to support the HTS facility. These results should be compared against the compound data provide by the synthesis laboratory, before the structures are stored in the library data base. Routine repetitive analysis of a representative set of compounds is advisable to monitor the status of the library over time. Contamination of the library can occur in several ways. Inattention to adequate tip-washing techniques, and in a microtiter plate, liquid format library, cross contamination from nearby wells, are the most common causes. However, contamination can occur from compounds extracted from the sample tube, the microtiter plate, the lid or sealer components, or from a combination of each. Studies are underway to investigate this and some information is already available from individual plate manufacturers. The larger companies, e.g., Becton Dickenson and Corning Costar, have undertaken such studies and information may be obtained by contacting their technical departments through the local technical representative. Some repository facilities require libraries held as dry films to be checked for chemical composition and concentration before use in a screening assay, since dissolution after drying may not be complete. This puts added strain on their analytical support groups as well as potentially slowing down the screening process.

Should a compound prove active, further analytical confirmation of purity can then be performed using more specialized techniques such as liquid chromatography/mass spectrometry (LC/MS). All of the data gathered about the composition of the library compounds should be recorded within the repository database for future reference.

2.2. Screening Facilities

HTS facilities vary in their charters and hence in their requirements. At one end of the spectrum, some HTS facilities are specific for a restricted type of assay format and at the other end are those facilities that have to accommodate any type of assay required by any therapeutic area within the company. It is generally easier to set up a facility for specific assays than to set one up to cover all eventualities. With a specific assay format, the physical plant of the facility can be arranged to give the optimum working environment for both people and instrumentation, whereas compromises have to be made for more complex and flexible installations.

2.3. Controlled Environment Screening

Many screening laboratories require that some of the instrumentation be able to be run in a sterile environment. Performance of cellular or microbiological assays requiring live cell seeding followed by addition of reagents and incubation are best carried out in completely sterile conditions. This is easier to arrange in a dedicated facility, as sterile areas can be arranged and maintained with specific parameters in mind and issues of equipment arrangement can be optimized. In a large open laboratory area or in a screening facility covering multiple assay types, this is more difficult to arrange. One solution to the sterility problem is to position individual pieces of automation beneath a series of ceiling mounted fans with high efficiency particulate air (HEPA) filters attached. Installations of this type are commercially available from companies manufacturing clean rooms but are also found as "in house" installed units in some facilities. A selection of address for companies specializing in this type of installation can be obtained from Cleanrooms.com of San Mateo, CA. (www.info@cleanrooms.com). The filtered fans provide a down flow curtain of "sterile air" which directs environmental contamination away from the equipment. These fans need to provide airflow of at least 90 cu ft/min when measured 6 inches from the fan outlet.

The best method for validating the efficiency of the air curtain is by electronic checking of the airflow velocity, followed by smoke testing, and is best done by a qualified external company. This monitoring does not preclude checks for surface contamination by airborne organisms. A simple check for viable organism levels can be performed by exposing unlidded petridishes, containing bacterial growth or fungal media, in the area under the running fans for a standard time period. The petri dishes should then be incubated and the growth level checked at 24 and 48 h (1).

Another solution to the problem of robotic sterility is to use some form of structural enclosure around the individual open automation units and have HEPA filtered air pumped in as an air curtain at approx 100 cu ft/min. Several manufacturers produce enclosures of this type, which have clear plastic walls and are capable of supporting the air-handling equipment on their roofs. In an open facility, use of these enclosures enables even bacterial and cell-culture screens to be done in close proximity to one another without worries of cross-contamination. This type of enclosure can also be used for odor containment in the chemical repository area by reversing the airflow and passing it through activated charcoal filters as it exits. Monitoring of the efficiency of the air-handling mechanisms in this type of enclosure is best contracted to an independent, biological hood certification company. In the absence of such a company, the airflow through the filters must be checked at least yearly using a simple airflow gauge, and the filters changed when the flow drops below 90 cu ft/min or after 3 yr, whichever comes first. Further details on the optimization of clean room systems can be obtained from standard texts *(2)*.

3. System Management and Support

The smooth running of a HTS facility requires attention not just to instrumentation, but also to the personnel who work in the facility. The performance of an HTS facility has more in common with a manufacturing process than with academia or research from which most of the screeners are recruited. The heavy emphasis on automation of repetitive tasks necessitates that engineering support be available at all times since the robotic complexity obviates the usual laboratory methods of self-support. It is not imperative that small HTS groups employ individual engineers if they feel that traditional equipment maintenance agreements and in-house expertise are adequate. Larger groups often find it necessary to have continuous engineering support and this comes either from internal company expertise or from specialist engineers hired directly into the screening group. Unless dedicated engineering support is very comprehensive, it is advisable that some form of service agreement be available for all the systems within a facility, so that highly specialized repairs can be done as quickly as possible. Most equipment vendors operate on a priority system for parts and supplies, and lack of a service contract often removes a company from the vendor's priority list. One attractive alternative to the previous solutions is for a service support contract to be developed with the instrument company providing the majority of the automation. This contract would ideally provide permanent on-site engineering support for the automation as well as blanket coverage for peripheral instrumentation attached to the robotics. Such contracts do exist and, although expensive, have proved very valuable to the companies able to implement them.

3.1. Routine System Management

Management of a multitasking HTS facility requires accurate scheduling of equipment use, which should be revisited on a regular basis. The method used for this must be easily understood and should include time for routine equipment maintenance as well the actual time the instrument is being used for assay runs during the day. A convenient time frame for the routine equipment use schedule is two weeks, but a master schedule is also needed to apportion assay campaigns during the year. Combined use of these two schedules allows for planning and information sharing between assay groups. Placing the routine schedule on a shared drive allows screeners to update equipment usage and improves the efficiency of the whole HTS facility.

3.2. Performance Tracking

One of the most important concepts in laboratory management is to understand the necessity of tracking performance *(3)*. This is done easily by the generation of "Key Indicator Tracking" data. A key indicator is a measure of a process of prime importance to the task under scrutiny. The workflow together with the key indicators required by a typical HTS facility is described in **Fig. 1**. Key indicators need to be in place for process and quality measurements when operating in the true high-performance work-team manner that has proved so successful in the manufacturing world *(4)*. Each key indicator measures progress towards a team-determined goal and is approved by the team members before implementation. These goals are revisited each year and are revised as necessary. The key indicators that have most relevance within the screening environment are the three quality measurements (Q1–Q3) and the three process measurements (P1–P3) described in **Fig. 1**. These indicators cover both instrument and personnel performance within the facility and are vital to ensure reliable performance and rapid resolution of problems. The key indicator data is determined by the team goals and collated into a visual form such as a graph by a designated team member. Most of the key indicators are updated weekly, with only two (P1 and Q4) being updated quarterly. All the indicator graphs are then displayed for the team's information at a central location within the screening facility.

3.3. Team Composition

The balance between the engineering, chemistry, and biological personnel in a screening group is peculiar to each individual company. Some companies have a preponderance of scientists relative to engineers, others have the reverse. Smaller groups with staffing problems often find it cost-effective to employ temporary personnel for the more routine portion of screening. All groups have the same difficulties in maintaining continuous quality control across all members. One effective method of making sure that continuous quality control occurs is to form a high-performance work team using cross-functional teams within the HTS unit. Teams within the unit have responsibility for defining the direction of a specific area within the overall unit and develop a work plan specific to their area. Examples of these teams could be an Assay Team, a Data Handling Team, and a Compound Team. Open communication channels need to be maintained within the overall HTS unit to ensure continuity. The efficiency of each team is monitored by quarterly feedback documents that are requested from each teams customers. In the case of HTS, customers are defined as groups, such as therapeutic areas, which accept data from the unit, or other teams within HTS. Within HTS, upward feedback is generated by the technical

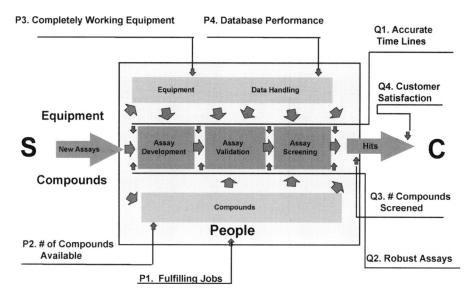

Fig. 1. HTS process chart: Diagrammatic representation of the indicators for performance (P) and quality (Q) used to measure the efficiency of the HTS system.

staff providing feedback on the supervisor's performance using the same basic system as for the customers of the whole team. All types of feedback forms are designed to provide constructive comments that can be acted on for future improvement and are generated quarterly. The forms can be completed anonymously and collated by someone outside of the group, preferably from human resources. An example is provided in Appendix 1. The data is then collated and graphs plotted showing progression towards the team's published goals. This data is reported out quarterly as the Q4 indicator. The HTS team holds annual workshops to analyze the previous year's results and to define the next year's challenges. An example of the graphs developed is shown in **Fig. 2**.

3.4. Equipment Performance Tracking

The function of the in-house engineering staff of an HTS facility is crucial. Their primary function is to provide engineering support to the robotics for reconfiguration or in a breakdown situation. An equally important part of their function is to oversee the records of each piece of equipment and to produce the historical information to enable the operators determine the equipment efficiency. When a new piece of instrumentation is received into the laboratory, all the manuals and software should be placed together in a well-defined

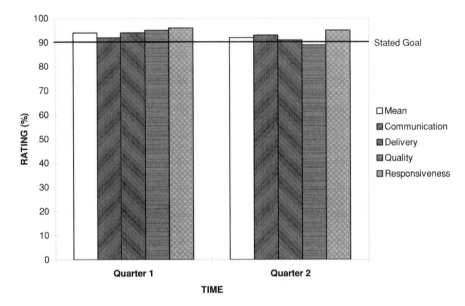

Fig. 2. Graphic representation of customer feedback measured over time identifying areas of potential improvement.

area for future reference. The first document, which needs to be written for every piece of equipment, is a description of the instrument and it's mode of action. This document need not be as detailed as a Standard Operating Procedure (SOP) required by manufacturing facilities, but detailed enough to provide easily followed instructions for casual users. In our hands these are dynamic documents that are updated regularly and are known as Current Best Approach documents or CBA's (*see* **Appendix 2**). In addition, each instrument has a laminated "cheat sheet" attached to it outlining the basic procedures of the instrument, such as how to switch it on and emergency procedures for shutting it down. The third document developed for each instrument is a logbook that is used for performance tracking. The information required held in the logbook is a historical, factual account of every procedure performed on the instrument, together with all the service reports for the equipment or its components. The operator must accurately fill in this record every time the equipment is used, even if the instrument performed perfectly. Correct use of this system allows slowly developing situations to be identified and dealt with before they become major problems. Basic laboratory general use equipment such as refrigerators, incubators, centrifuges, and hand-held pipetting units should be included in this performance documentation, with practical adjustments made to the paper work (e.g., no "cheat sheets" for individual hand-held pipettors).

There are several widely used systems for tracking instrument performance, varying from completely manual to fully computerized. The major problem with any tracking system is that it usually relies on human introduction of information. The simplest method of information gathering is the previously mentioned logbook. This is attached to each instrument or workstation and into which information is entered as each run is performed. Transfer of data from this logbook to a spreadsheet for historical tracking is time-consuming and error-prone. One of the most efficient methods is for each instrument's 'run program' to have an electronic spreadsheet attached to it that must be completed before any run data can be archived. The information required by this spread sheet is identical to that required in the logbook method and a similar format can be devised. The collected data is then automatically downloaded into an historical data file and stored. Currently there are no commercial programs able to do this and those in use are site specific. An example of the basic data required maintaining historical tracking of instrument reliability is to be found in **Fig. 3**. This is an example of the instrument-reliability graph posted as HTS key indicator P3. Recording runs completed both with and without operator intervention enable distinctions to be made between simple malfunctions and those requiring engineering intervention. On multitasking systems differentiation between errors of software and peripheral hardware are often picked up in this manner. A similar graph can be produced from the electronic data-acquisition system should that be available. The results from either method must be reviewed on a regular basis and remedial action taken if necessary.

4. Examples of Requirements for Maintenance Programs
4.1. Pipetting and Dispensing Equipment

Routine checking of all pipetting and dispensing equipment for accuracy is one of the primary requirements of any HTS maintenance program. Any valid quality-control program should require all pipetting and dispensing units, both manual and automated, to be checked independently at least twice yearly. This procedure can be performed either in house or by a reputable outside contractor. All calibration records should be kept by both the contractor and the owner laboratory as a safeguard in case of future problems. In all cases the operator should be aware that the quality of the disposable tips used with any type of aspiration pipetting or dispensing unit has direct bearing on the reliability of the whole system. At no time should tips be used that are not recommended by the equipment manufacturer. Some tip manufacturers apply strict quality controls to their manufacturing processes and statistical details of the manufacturing batches can be obtained if requested. Common variations in pipetting accuracy are blocked tips or dispensing head mandrels, failure of the dispense

OPERATIONAL EQUIPMENT

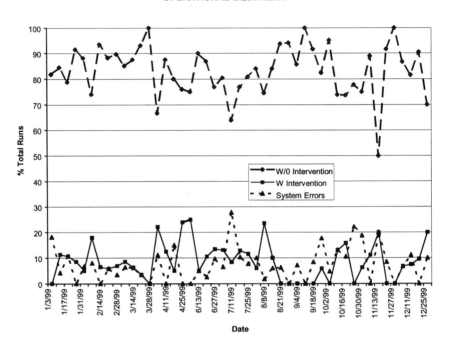

Fig. 3. An example of historical reliability data and error charting for a routine HTS laboratory.

mechanism itself, and lack of attention to the viscosity of the liquid being pipetted. Maintenance of peristaltic dispensing units also requires similar dispensing volume validation. Most dispensing heads on this type of equipment are calibrated during manufacture and need rechecking during use to confirm their performance efficiency. They should be replaced at regular intervals or when performance efficiency begins to deteriorate. It is considered good practice to run check plates of each liquid handling device prior to each assay run to prevent potential pipetting errors. There are two commonly used methods for checking the reliability of any type of dispensing tool. The first is a spectrophotometric method using a colored solution and is of most use for pipetting units with capacities above 50 μL and thus is used for 96-well microtiter plates. The microtiter plates used for this procedure must have flat-bottomed wells and be as optically clear as possible to cut down on optical-reader distortion. Some laboratories prefer to use glass microtiter plates for this procedure. The optical density of the dispensed liquid in each well is read at the peak wavelength of the chosen dye. This procedure can be performed with food coloring, which is easily obtained, and the spectrum of which can easily be determined on any scanning spectrophotometer. The second method employs fluorescene, which is used for much smaller pipetting volumes and requires the use of a fluorescence spectrophotometer with a 490 nm excitation filter and a 520 nm emission filter to read the results *(5)*. Solid black or white microtiter plates should be used with the fluorescence technique to reduce the well to well cross-talk and to obtain the most sensitive signal. The concentration of the dyes in both cases should be adjusted to give values within the center of the readers sensitivity range so maximum accuracy is obtained.

All dispensing is into microtiter plates and the results read on microtiter plate spectrophotometers or fluorometers, which allow visualization of the results in a plate format, thus easily isolating problems with individual mandrels and/or tips. Analysis of the results from these tests should give the operator the mean well volume with the standard deviation. Two other useful parameters are the standard deviation of the rows and columns across the plate. If there is a suspicion of problems with disposable tips then several iterations of the method should be performed to check the reproducibility across a series of tip loads. The same method can be used for 384-well dispensing units and the same calculations performed. An alternate method of reading is to use the weight of the microtiter plate before and after dispensing a fixed volume of liquid. This does not enable checks to be made on individual mandrels but just records the total volume dispensed. If the pipetting head is found to be defective, a document recording all the observed parameters should accompany the freshly cleaned head when it is returned to the manufacturer for refurbishing.

4.2. Detection Equipment

The detection equipment found in a screening laboratory depends on the type of assays done by that facility. Usually equipment for fluorescence, spectrophotometric, luminescence, and radiometric measurements are all required. Detection units, which are automation-friendly, are readily available for each measurement type and it is advisable to purchase multiples of the same type of detector if finances allow. Use of identical equipment permits assays entering screening to be developed using the same parameters as will be required when they are transferred to full-scale automation. This is a simple method if using a modular robotic system, but often difficult if custom designed systems are used. A common misconception about detection instruments is that identical models will perform in identical fashion. This is not necessarily the case since the majority of detection equipment still uses photomultiplier tubes (PMTs) and these can vary significantly from instrument to instrument. This misconception becomes very obvious when several instruments with unmatched PMTs are used to perform fluorescent polarization. In some cases the software can be manipulated to "balance" the results of a single assay between differing instruments to give consistent results. " Balancing" should always be carried out with the knowledge of the instrument manufacturer since some parameter changes could lead to confusion when a routine service engineer is called in for unrelated problems. This balancing process has to be repeated every time a lamp or PMT is changed. Misunderstandings due to lack of adequate operator training often result in little attention being paid to the type and quality of the filters used within detectors. This is of great importance in fluorescence assays using several endpoint detectors in one assay or on one robotic unit where it is imperative that all filters be identical to ensure data integrity. Information on standard filters is usually easily obtained since most companies provide details of the filter parameters in their instrument manuals. Lists of the filters used within individual instruments should be kept in the instrument logbook and alteration of the filter profiles restricted. Alteration of filter positions within an instrument must be also noted in the instrument logbook and software. Failure to do this will result in measurement errors when the wrong filter is used. Routine checking of filter sensitivity should be carried out if at all possible. Microtiter plates containing stable fluorescent indicators can be obtained for this procedure and checking the results of these plates over time will give an indication of the reliability of the detector light path.

End-point detection in luminescent and radioactive assays is usually performed with the same instrumentation. These instruments were primarily designed for radioactive assays but were found to be suitable for luminescent measurements. Checking of this instrumentation for background and normalization must be done on a regular basis using the instructions provided by the manufacturer. The use of injection or "flash" luminescence has resulted in the introduction of reagent injection units into some radioactive detectors. These injection units are rugged but require regular cleaning methods to be in place to prevent clogging of the liquid-handling system. Since there are routinely only one or two injection ports per unit, it is a relatively trivial task for the operators to perform at the end of each run. One method that can be used is the fluorescence-dye technique outlined in the liquid-handling maintenance section followed by repeated flushing of the injection system to remove all contamination (*see* **Subheading 4.1.**).

In this discussion of the detection equipment only common instrumentation has been mentioned. There are many different manufacturers with a variety of alternate methods of detection, all of which provide some improvement for a specific assay type. If all available assay types are supported, it can result in a large number of differing designs of detection units being needed within the screening facility. This scenario is expensive to implement and difficult to maintain. To address this situation some manufacturers have developed equipment with the ability to detect several different end-points, e.g., combined fluorescence and spectrophotometric readers. Many of these combination detector designs have a bias towards one of the detection mechanisms and thus need to be carefully evaluated before purchase.

4.3. Developmental Equipment

In addition to the robotic instrumentation within an HTS facility, the equipment used for development of assays and for development of novel screening technology has to be accommodated. In an ideal situation the dispensing and detection instrumentation required for development of potential screening assays should duplicate the equipment that will be used in the final automation systems in order to simplify cross validation. Such luxury is not possible for most laboratories and so accommodations have to be made that nearly always delay the speed of the screens. The equipment used for development of new screening technology is often from smaller vendors without adequate engineering support systems and no published methods for accuracy checking. In these cases, it is advisable that the operator develop both training and maintenance documentation for each novel item. Both of these types of equipment must also be regularly serviced and calibrated in line with the larger units.

4.4. Computer Maintenance

Nearly all of the equipment in a screening laboratory uses personal computers (PCs) to control both the robotics and to handle the generated data. PCs are powerful tools when operating properly, but they can cripple productivity when they fail. Laboratory PCs frequently have specialized hardware and software requirements dictated by the vendor of the equipment the computer is connected to. End users can save time and money by following a few basic guidelines in helping to maintain their lab computers.

When a new PC enters into the lab keep all the manuals and software together for future reference. This is especially important when there are numerous PCs in the lab. If serious problems develop in the future, one of the information technology (IT) professionals may need the specific disk or manual that came with the computer to troubleshoot and fix it. A logbook for each computer should be set up when the computer is received. The model and serial numbers must be recorded in it along with date and vendor. Each time the hardware is upgraded or new software is installed or modified the alterations to the system must be added to the logbook. This history can be very helpful when trying to troubleshoot problems.

A startup disk or emergency-repair disk should be made and updated at any time changes are made to the system. It's a good idea to run a check disc or utilities program once a week and to "Defrag" once a month. These utilities can often catch and fix minor problems before they turn into big ones. Old, unused log files, temp files, etc., that gradually fill up and slow down your hard drive (HD) should be cleaned out at the same time.

Statistically, the HD is one of the most likely hardware components to fail. When the hard drive fails, not only is all data lost but so is the operating system, application programs, and custom settings, methods, and tweaks, sometimes the hardest to recover. It is preferable to perform full HD backups for all critical computer systems. Backing up can be done to an outside server or independently to a hardware storage system. There are two parts to providing an independent backup: first the backup software and then the hardware storage device. If the HD fails and requires replacing, the same backup software can be used to restore (copy back) the entire contents of the original HD to the new one, complete with all custom settings, etc.

4.5. Data Management

Data files from detectors should be moved to an independent server or personal computer at the earliest opportunity. Reliance on the detector internal-storage system can occasionally lead to loss of data files due to mistakes from different operators using the same equipment. Backing up and general management of assay data files should be the responsibility of the screener in charge of that assay since "ownership" is a potent force in the efficient performance of a screen. Validation of data-handling packages is a complex procedure and should also be included in the continuous monitoring off a high-performance facility (*6*).

All data should be backed up on a daily or "each run" basis to minimize loss in event of an accident. The most efficient method for data handling is "real time data acquisition and calculation," which is available only to those screening groups having adequate IT support. Lack of foresight by some groups in the past has resulted in companies having data-handling packages, which have very rapidly become too small to handle all their requirements. When a data-handling package is purchased it should ideally be very flexible and have the ability to interface with all other software packages used within the screening group, chemistry, and the therapeutic areas. The ability of all groups to access and enter data into the same linked system cuts down on errors and misunderstandings and eases data mining. This type of system is always large and requires extensive IT support to maintain it reliably and the cost and requirements for its upkeep can make it an unattractive option for some facilities.

5. Conclusion

It is hoped that this chapter will provide both new and experienced screeners with fresh insights into the complexity of maintaining an efficient HTS facility and will provide a basis for improving the work processes within all screening facilities. Continuing improvement to the processes will result in even greater efficiency and reliability resulting in faster and hopefully better, identification of new drug entities that will result in benefits for all.

References

1. *Microorganisms in Clean Rooms, Standard IEST-RP-CC023-1.* (1993) Institute of Environmental Sciences and Technology (IEST), 940, E. Northwest Hwy, Mt. Prospect, IL 60056.
2. Liptak, B. G., (1998) *Optimization of Industrial Unit Operations.* CRC Press, Boca Raton, FL.
3. Shewhart, W. A. and Deming, W. E. (1990) *Statistical Method from the Viewpoint of Quality Control.* Dover Publications Inc., Mineola, NY.
4. Graham Brown, M. G. (1997) *Baldridge Award Winning Quality.* Productivity Press Inc., Portland, OR.
5. *CCS Packard/PlateTrak Service manual revision* (2000) Packard Bioscience, 2841, Lomita Blvd, Torrance, CA 90505.
6. Lewis, W. E. (2000) *Software Testing and Continuous Quality Improvement.* CRC Press, Boca Raton, FL.

Appendix 1

EMPLOYEE SATISFACTION INDEX

Appraising (Name): _____

Your Name: _____ Date: _____

	GRADE	SCORE
A	Total Customer Satisfaction	>90%
B	Customer Generally Satisfied	70-89%
C	Customer Generally Dissatisfied	40-69%
D	Total Customer Dissatisfaction	<40%

* If Scoring is rated "B" or less, please explain your reason so that improvements can be made.

** Please give an exact numerical score as well as a letter grade.

	GRADE	SCORE
Communication: Use of basic principles, effective method established for two-way verbal and written message or instructions, and timely communication relevant to helping you do your daily work.		
Delivery: Timeliness, keeps promises, facilitates work flow, helps eliminate barriers to help you do your job.		
Quality: Provides quality product and/or service (i.e., accurate information), provides ideas, consistency, and clear priorities, communicates and follows up on short- and long-term career development needs.		
Responsiveness: Exhibits courtesy and professionalism, provides appropriate and timely feedback and advice resulting in total employee satisfaction.		

Comments:

_____

_____

_____

Appendix 2

CURRENT BEST APPROACH

High Throughput Screening Laboratory

Date	Equipment/Instrumentation	Page
		1/

Type of Instrument
Operation, Calibration, Maintenance and Identification

I. SCOPE: This CBA describes the general procedures to be followed by users of the instrument. General operating procedures, validation procedures and maintenance procedures will be described.

II. REFERENCES: Often reference to the instrument manual

III. COMPONENTS/PERIPHERALS: A complete list of instrument components if modular, including computer.

IV. RESPONSIBILITIES:

PERSONNEL	RESPONSIBILITIES
Scientist	For running, for repairs etc.

V. SPECIFIC PROCEDURES: What it can be used for.

VI. SUITABILITY: Description of suitability of instrument for task.

A. Operation	Detailed practical documentation.
B. Calibration	Specific protocol for instrument.
C. Safety Issues	Specific to the instrument
D. Documentation and Record Keeping	Where kept and in what format.
E. Identification and labeling	Model, serial number and other identification.

VI. ATTACHMENTS: Any other documentation.

Approval Signatures: Date:

_____   _____

_____   _____

Author: Date:

_____   _____

Index

Global screening database, 130–131
Glucokinase
  activators, 164
Glucolipsin A, 164
  structure, 165
Glucolipsin B, 164
  structure, 165
Glutathione antibodies, 36
GPCRs. *See* G-protein coupled
    receptors (GPCRs)
G-protein coupled receptors
    (GPCRs), 6, 7, 34, 108
  and HTS, 2–4
Graphical User Interface (GUI), 138
  style, 179
GST-Rb152-strep tag
  expression and purification,
      67–68, 70
  phosphorylation, 73
GUI, 138, 179

H

Hamilton Co., 170
Hard event times, 179
HEPA filters, 232
Heuristic scheduling, 179
High-content screens, 114
High efficiency particulate air
    (HEPA) filters, 232
High Performance Serial Bus
    (HPSB), 180
High throughput screening assays
  design and implementation, 1–27
High throughput screening (HTS)
  continuing trends, 215
  data, 45–47
  description, 1
  equipment requirements, 230–233
    chemical repository, 230–231

controlled environment
    screening, 232–233
  screening facilities, 231
  issues, 42–45
  maintenance program
      requirements, 237–241
    computer maintenance, 241
    detection equipment, 239–241
    developmental equipment, 241
    pipetting and dispensing
        equipment, 237–239
  manipulation and maintenance,
      229–243
  process, 1–2
  process chart, 235
  system management and support,
      233–237
    equipment performance
        tracking, 235–237
    performance tracking, 234
    routine management, 233
    team composition, 234–235
High throughput screening
    (HTS)workstations
  introduced since 1998
    manufacturers, models, and
        types, 211–212
Homogeneous mix-and-read
    formats, 5
Homogenous time-resolved
    fluorescence resonance energy
    transfer (HTR-FRET), 66
HPSB, 180
HTR-FRET, 66
HTS. *See* High throughput screening
    (HTS)
Hudson Control Group
  address, 190
Humidity, 118
  chemical repository, 230
Hydrazide, 89